Measurement of

Cardiac
Function

CRC Press
METHODS IN THE LIFE SCIENCES

Gerald D. Fasman - Advisory Editor
Brandeis University

Series Overview

Methods in Biochemistry
John Hershey
Department of Biological Chemistry
University of California

Cellular and Molecular Neuropharmacology
Joan M. Lakoski
Department of Pharmacology
Penn State University

Research Methods for Inbred Laboratory Mice
John P. Sundberg
The Jackson Laboratory
Bar Harbor, Maine

Methods in Neuroscience
Sidney A. Simon
Department of Neurobiology
Duke University

Joseph M. Corless
Department of Cell Biology,
Neurobiology and Ophthalmology
Duke University

Methods in Pharmacology
John H. McNeill
Professor and Dean
Faculty of Pharmaceutical Science
The University of British Columbia

Methods in Signal Transduction
Joseph Eichberg, Jr.
Department of Biochemical and Biophysical Sciences
University of Houston

Methods in Toxicology
Edward J. Massaro
Senior Research Scientist
National Health and Environmental Effects Research Laboratory
Research Triangle Park, North Carolina

CRC Press
METHODS IN PHARMACOLOGY

John H. McNeill
Faculty of Pharmaceutical Sciences
The University of British Columbia
Vancouver, B.C. CANADA

The *CRC Press Methods in Pharmacology Series* provides the reader with a step-by-step approach to each of the classical and up-to-date methods and presents techniques in a clear and concise format. Topics covering all aspects of pharmacology are being reviewed for publication.

Published Titles

Biochemical Techniques in the Heart, John H. McNeill
Measurement of Cardiac Function, John H. McNeill
Measurement of Cardiovascular Function, John H. McNeill

Forthcoming Titles

Methods in Cardiac Electrophysiology

Measurement of
Cardiac
Function

Edited by

John H. McNeill, Ph.D.

Department of Pharmaceutical Sciences
University of British Columbia
Vancouver, Canada

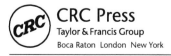

CRC Press
Taylor & Francis Group
Boca Raton London New York

CRC Press is an imprint of the
Taylor & Francis Group, an **informa** business

CRC Press
Taylor & Francis Group
6000 Broken Sound Parkway NW, Suite 300
Boca Raton, FL 33487-2742

© 1997 by Taylor & Francis Group, LLC
CRC Press is an imprint of Taylor & Francis Group, an Informa business

No claim to original U.S. Government works

ISBN 13: 978-0-8493-3332-3 (pbk)

Visit the Taylor & Francis Web site at
http://www.taylorandfrancis.com

and the CRC Press Web site at
http://www.crcpress.com

Library of Congress Cataloging-in-Publication Data

Measurement of cardiac function / edited by John H. McNeill.
    p.   cm. — (CRC Press methods in the life sciences. Methods
in pharmacology)
    Includes bibliographical references and index.
    ISBN 0-8493-3332-6
    1. Heart — Research — Laboratory manuals.   2. Heart function tests —
-Laboratory manuals.   I. McNeill, John H.   II. Series.
    [DNLM: 1. Heart — physiology.   WG202M484 1996]
QP112.4.M43 1996
612.1'7'0724--dc20
DNLM/DLC
for Library of Congress

                                                                    96-31525
                                                                      CIP

Cover Design: Denise Craig

Library of Congress Card Number 96-31525

Dedication

To my wife Sharon and my daughters Sandy and Laurie.
You are always there for me.

Preface

The books in this series have been conceived as a trilogy on "Methods in Experimental Cardiology" and represent the only texts providing a detailed description of the main techniques used in understanding physiological and pathophysiological cardiovascular regulation. In order to enhance the effectiveness and readability, the work has been divided into three volumes. Volume 1, *Measurement of Cardiac Function*, includes chapters on The Langendorff Heart, The Isolated Working Heart, Isolated Papillary Muscle Preparations, Isolated Atrial Muscle Preparations, *In Vivo* Measurements of Cardiac Function, and Isolated Ventricle Measurements. Volume 2 is entitled *Measurement of Cardiovascular Function* and includes chapters on The Lipid Perfused Heart, Metabolic Measurements in the Heart, Models of Arrhythmia, Techniques for Arterial Blood Pressure Measurement, and Models of Experimental Hypertension. Volume 3, *Biochemical Techniques in the Heart*, deals with Preparation of SR, Preparation of Sarcolemma, Measurement of Sodium-Calcium Exchange, Measurement of Sodium-Potassium ATPase, Molecular Assessment of the Sodium-Potassium ATPase, Measurement of Sodium-Hydrogen Exchange, and Preparation of Cardiomyocytes.

Each chapter has been peer-reviewed and carefully edited in order to provide an up-to-date, comprehensive, practical, portable, and accessible guide to the main experimental techniques used in examining *in vivo, ex vivo*, and *in vitro* cardiac function in animals. The text answers a long-felt need and represents the contribution of an outstanding group of authors who provide the cardiovascular audience with the "*recipe*" of the techniques: setting up the method, starting material required and their procurement, the "do's and don'ts," troubleshooting and resolution, sample data, spreadsheets and calculations, and modifications and applicability.

With multiple flowcharts, diagrams, and actual photographs, these simple and straightforward texts will serve both as a research reference and a bench guide for the cardiac physiologist, pharmacologist, biochemist, and trainee and will hopefully save hours of precious research time.

John H. McNeill, Ph.D.
Professor and Dean
Faculty of Pharmaceutical Sciences
The University of British Columbia

The Editor

John H. McNeill, Ph.D., is Professor of Pharmacology and Toxicology and Dean of the Faculty of Pharmaceutical Sciences at The University of British Columbia in Vancouver, Canada.

Dr. McNeill graduated in 1960 from the University of Alberta with a B.Sc., (Pharm) degree. He obtained his M.Sc. from the same institution 2 years later and his Ph.D. in Pharmacology at the University of Michigan in 1967.

Dr. McNeill is a member of the Pharmacological Society of Canada, the American Society for Pharmacology and Experimental Therapeutics, the Western Pharmacology Society, the International Society for Heart Research, the Association of Faculties of Pharmacy, American Pharmaceutical Association, Sigma Xi, American Diabetes Association, Canadian Diabetes Association and Canadian Pharmaceutical Association. Dr. McNeill served on the Council and as President of the Canadian Pharmacology Society and the Western Pharmacology Society and on the Council of the North American Section and the international body of the International Society for Heart Research. He has served on and chaired many Canadian national research committees for the MRC, Canadian Heart and Stroke Foundation, Canadian Diabetes Association, and the PMAC–Health Research Foundation. He currently serves on the jury for the prestigious Prix Galien Award.

Dr. McNeill has received a number of awards for his research including the Upjohn Award (Canadian Pharmacology Society), McNeil Award (Association of Faculties of Pharmacy of Canada), and the Jacob Biely Award and Killam Award from The University of British Columbia. He has been an MRC Visiting Professor at a number of Canadian universities and at Montpellier University in France.

Dr. McNeill has presented numerous invited lectures in North America, Europe and Japan and has published over 350 manuscripts, reviews and book chapters. His current major research interests are diabetes-induced cardiomyopathy, hyperinsulinemia and hypertension, glucose-lowering agents, and mechanisms of action of insulin.

Contributors

Joseph M. Capasso, Ph.D.
Division of Cardio-Renal Drugs
U.S. Food and Drug Administration
Rockville, Maryland

Ahmad B. Fawzi, Ph.D.
Schering-Plough Research Institute
Kenilworth, New Jersey

E.S. Hayes, Ph.D.
Department of Pharmacology and
  Therapeutics
The University of British Columbia
Vancouver, British Columbia, Canada

Tony Hebden, Ph.D.
Department of Chemistry
Simon Fraser University
Burnaby, British Columbia. Canada

Thane G. Maddaford, B.Sc.
Ion Transport Laboratory
Division of Cardiovascular Sciences
St. Boniface General Hospital
  Research Center
Winnipeg, Manitoba, Canada

Hamid Massaeli, B.Sc.
Ion Transport Laboratory
Division of Cardiovascular Sciences
St. Boniface General Hospital
  Research Center
Winnipeg, Manitoba, Canada

Grant N. Pierce, Ph.D.
Ion Transport Laboratory
Division of Cardiovascular Sciences
St. Boniface General Hospital
  Research Center
Winnipeg, Manitoba, Canada

Michael K. Pugsley, Ph.D.
Department of Pharmacology and
  Therapeutics
The University of British Columbia
Vancouver, British Columbia, Canada

Robert L. Rodgers, Ph.D.
Department of Pharmacology and
  Toxicology
University of Rhode Island
Kingston, Rhode Island

Michael J.A. Walker, Ph.D.
Department of Pharmaceutical Sciences
University of Briitish Columbia
Vancouver, British Columbia, Canada

Acknowledgments

I would like to thank Jeff Hillier who first discussed the idea for these books with me many years ago and Paul Petralia who arm-wrestled me into finding the time to actually go ahead and bring the project to fruition. Two of my graduate students, Margaret Cam and Subodh Verma reviewed all of the book chapters from the perspective of a graduate student. Subodh was my strong right arm in badgering authors, helping me edit, and ensuring that everything was done properly. To him, I owe a tremendous debt.

Contents

Chapter 1

The Langendorff Heart

Ahmad B. Fawzi

Contents

1. Introduction

The Langendorff heart preparation is one of the earliest models of an isolated organ, used by physiologists and pharmacologists to investigate function and the effect of different agents on an isolated tissue. This preparation was first described by O. Langendorff in 1895.[1] The procedure is based on perfusing an isolated heart through the aorta (retrograde) with an oxygenated physiological buffer. The resulting retrograde perfusion pressure closes the aortic valve, facilitating the perfusion of the coronary blood vessels located at the

0-8493-3332-6/97/$0.00+$.50
© 1997 by CRC Press, Inc.

base of the aorta. As the heart is a highly vascularized organ, the physiological buffer eventually gains access to all cells within the heart. Since the heart requires a steady supply of oxygen and metabolic energy for its normal functioning, it is crucial to rapidly extract the organ from the chest cavity without an episode of ischemia, prevent occlusion of the coronary arteries with blood clots, and rapidly supply the organ with a highly oxygenated physiological buffer.

Through a century of utilization of the Langendorff heart, there have been numerous modifications of the original Langendorff apparatus, an evolution which was inevitable as advances in technology enhanced our ability to build better and more reliable devices. In this chapter, the basic principles and methods required for preparing a reliable Langendorff heart are described.

2. Applications

Considering that ventricular muscle is highly vascularized, inotropic agents perfused into the heart rapidly gain access to all ventricular muscle cells, leading to a greater sensitivity of the preparation to perfused agents. Hence, the Langendorff heart preparation is ideal for studying the concentration-dependent effects of positive and negative inotropic agents on cardiac contractility.[2] Agents that increase the force of ventricular muscle contraction (positive inotropic agents) increase intraventricular pressure and the contractility index $+dP/dt_{max}$, while agents that reduce the force of contraction (negative inotropic agents) reduce intraventricular pressure and $+dP/dt_{max}$. An example of the effect of such agents on the guinea pig heart is shown in Figure 1.[3] Additionally, as some inotropic agents alter heart rate and coronary flow, the Langendorff heart preparation described here eliminates limitations induced by these factors. For example, as negative inotropic agents reduce ventricular function, aortic perfusion pressure is diminished, leading to cessation of coronary flow and heart failure due to ischemia. In the Langendorff heart, coronary perfusion pressure and coronary flow are independent of ventricular muscle function. This is in contrast to the working heart model, where aortic perfusion pressure is dependent on left ventricular function.[4] Finally, a fixed balloon size in the present preparation ensures measurement of isometric tension at an optimal muscle fiber length.

In addition to the above-described physiological and pharmacological measurements, the Langendorff heart preparation has also been widely used in the study of metabolic changes brought about by ventricular contraction and relaxation.[5] Additionally, the effect of ischemia and hypoxia on cardiac metabolism and function has also been studied using the Langendorff isolated heart.[6,7] The preparation could also be utilized for evaluating the effect of different agents which act on coronary blood vessels. For this purpose, the heart is perfused under a constant pressure from a buffer reservoir placed at a constant height above the heart, and coronary flow is monitored by measuring

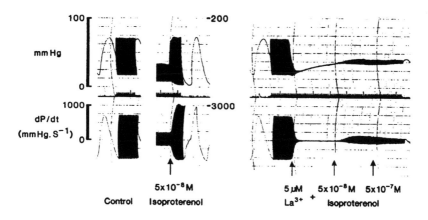

Figure 1
Effect of isoproterenol and lanthanum on contractility of the guinea pig heart. The figure shows original tracings of a Langendorff preparation of an adult guinea pig heart perfused with Hepes buffer containing 1.8 mM calcium. The upper part of the tracing shows intraventricular pressure of the left ventricle and the bottom part shows the first derivative of the pressure curve (dP/dt) recorded simultaneously. Following 45 min equilibration with Hepes buffer, the heart was perfused with the maximum effective concentration of isoproterenol (5 × 10^{-8} M). Note that sensitivity of the recording was altered to fully record the increase in intraventricular pressure and dP/dt induced by isoproterenol treatment. Isoproterenol was rapidly washed out and perfusion was continued with Hepes buffer for 45 min. Following washout with buffer, basal contractility returned to its initial control level. The heart was then perfused with 5 µM lanthanum followed by the same concentration of lanthanum plus 5 × 10^{-8} and 5 × 10^{-7} M isoproterenol. (From Fawzi, A.B. and McNeill, J.H., *Can. J. Physiol. Pharmacol.*, 63, 1106, 1985. With permission.)

buffer flow rate through the heart.[8] Alternatively, the heart is perfused with buffer at a constant flow rate and aortic perfusion pressure is used as an index of constriction or dilatation of coronary blood vessels.[9]

3. Methods

3.1. The Langendorff Apparatus

The key elements for successful operation of a Langendorff heart are (a) uniform flow of buffer at a constant pressure; (b) constant temperature of the perfused buffer; and (c) continous oxygenation of the buffer. Figure 2 shows the basic design of the apparatus. To supply buffer to the heart, one can simply place the buffer container at a height to provide a 60 mm Hg pressure to the base of the aorta. An alternative method is to use a peristaltic pump (Pharmacia Biotech Pump P-1) such that buffer flow is adjusted to provide the desired perfusion pressure (8 to 9 ml/min). Buffer should reach the heart at a constant temperature ranging from 30 to 37°C (Proportional Temperature Controller YSI Model 72; Fisher Scientific). Some investigators prefer perfusing the heart

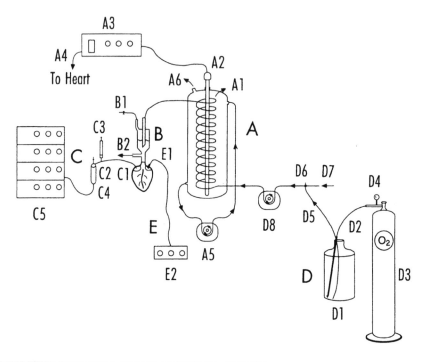

Figure 2

The figure shows a schematic model of the Langendorff apparatus. The major parts of the apparatus are labeled alphabetically, whereas components are marked with an alphabet letter followed by a number. **A.** *Jacketed glass water bath.* Buffer is pumped into the bath through a coiled glass tube (**A1**). A porcelain heating element (**A2**) is placed in the center of the bath to maintain the water in the bath at the desired temperature. The heating element is connected to a regulated proportional power supply (**A3**). Amount of power supplied to the heating element is determined by the set point on the power supply and the feedback obtained from temperature of the heart detected by a flexible temperature probe (**A4**). The probe can either be placed inside the right atrium or water bath (via inlet **A6**). To ensure an even temperature throughout the bath, distilled water inside the bath is circulated by a peristaltic pump (**A5**). A large volume of water in the bath (500 to 700 ml) is required to prevent temperature fluctuations. **B.** *Air bubble trap.* This device, made of glass, plays a crucial role in preventing air bubbles from entering the heart. It is supplied with two outlets: **B1**, connected to a Tygon tube and a two-way valve to release excess air and regulate buffer level in the trap, and **B2**, which is connected to a pressure transducer for monitoring buffer pressure. **C.** *Latex balloon.* The balloon, which is inserted into the heart, is connected to the end of a polyethylene tube (**C1**) attached to a three-way valve (**C2**), a 2-ml syringe (**C3**), a pressure transducer (**C4**), and polygraph (**C5**). **D.** *Physiological buffer and peristaltic pump.* Buffer is placed in a suitable container (**D1**) and is continuously supplied with 95% CO_2/5%O_2 through an aerator (**D2**) connected to gas tank (**D3**) and a regulator (**D4**). Buffer is drawn from the container through a Tygon tube (**D5**) connected to a three-way valve (**D6**). The valve is connected to a second Tygon tube (**D7**) for perfusion of buffer containing the test compound. A regulated peristaltic pump (**D8**) is used to pump the buffer to the heart through the jacketed bath. **E.** *Stimulator and electrode.* The heart is stimulated at double its threshold voltage through platinum electrodes (**E1**) placed on the surface of the right atria. Pulse stimulation is provided by a stimulator (**E2**).

at 37°C. However, a lower temperature of 30°C allows for a longer operation of the heart with a consistent heart function. A constant temperature is achieved by passing the buffer through a jacketed water bath (diameter 7 cm; height 17 cm) just before it enters the heart. The temperature is set at around 2°C higher than the desired temperature, which is measured by placing a thermometer at the end of the aortic cannula. The buffer should be aerated continuously with 95% O_2 to 5% CO_2. To avoid the transmission of air bubbles into the coronary blood vessels, a bubble trap should be placed above the heart. Hence, buffer leaving the jacketed coil flows into the bubble trap before reaching the heart. The trap is connected to a pressure transducer to monitor perfusion pressure of the buffer before it enters the heart. It also contains a release valve to release excess air bubbles in the trap.

For monitoring ventricular pressure, some investigators insert a needle connected to a pressure transducer (GRASS Instruments) into the base of the left ventricle. To monitor isometric tension developed by the left ventricle, a small latex balloon filled with saline and connected to a pressure transducer is inserted into the left ventricle via a small incision made in the left atrium. The balloon is made from thin latex material such as the tip of a nonlubricated condom. The balloon is connected to a 1- or 2-ml syringe filled with saline to adjust its size. The balloon is deflated prior to insertion into the left ventricle. Following careful insertion, the balloon is gradually inflated with saline so that it fills the left ventricular cavity. In this manner, the left ventricle is stretched to its optimum size, and it will function in an isovolumic mode as the size of the balloon is kept constant throughout the experiment.

3.2. Buffers

A modified Krebs-Henseleit[10] bicarbonate buffer (pH 7.4) equilibrated with 95% O_2:5% CO_2 is used to perfuse the heart. Final concentrations of constituents in the buffer are (in mM): NaCl, 118; KCl, 4.7; $CaCl_2$, 1.8; $MgSO_4$, 1.2; KH_2PO_4, 1.2; $NaHCO_3$, 25; and glucose, 11.2, made in distilled water. Tenfold concentrated stock solutions of NaCl and 100-fold concentrated stock solutions of KCl, $CaCl_2$, $MgSO_4$, and KH_2PO_4 are recommended. Buffer is prepared fresh on the day of the experiment by mixing the above stock solutions to obtain the recommended final concentrations of all agents. Glucose and $NaHCO_3$ are weighed and added on the day of the experiment. The buffer is then continuously equilibrated with 95% O_2:5% CO_2 for 1 h to saturate buffer with O_2, maintain pH at 7.4, and prevent precipitation of calcium salts. To prevent precipitation of calcium salts, the above mixing and gassing is recommended before addition of $NaHCO_3$.

Hepes buffer (pH 7.4) can also be used when testing the effects of high concentrations of calcium and metal ions on the heart. Buffer composition is (in mM): NaCl, 140; KCl, 4.5; $MgCl_2$, 1.2; $CaCl_2$, 1.8; Hepes, 3; and glucose, 11.2. Buffer pH is adjusted to 7.4 and gassed with 100% O_2. As described above, concentrated stock solutions can be prepared, except that Hepes and glucose are weighed and dissolved in the buffer on the day of experiment.

All agents to be tested on the heart should be dissolved in these physiological buffers, which are continously gassed throughout the experiment.

3.3.   Preparation of the Heart

Animals are injected with heparin (1000 U/kg, i.p.) 20 min before initiation of the experiment. To attain surgical anesthesia, halothane (Fluothane, Ayerst Laboratories) can be used for smaller animals like rats and guinea pigs. Animals are placed in a glass jar saturated with halothane until they demonstrate muscle relaxation, slow breathing, and absence of reflexes. For larger animals like rabbits, pentobarbital sodium (MTC Pharmaceuticals) can be given i.v. into the marginal ear vein. To open the thoracic cavity, lift skin just below the rib cage with forceps and using sharp surgical scissors, remove fur and make a transverse cut through the abdominal cavity. All subsequent steps following opening of the abdominal cavity should be carried out in the shortest time possible to prevent myocardial ischemia. Cut through the diaphragm and make two lateral incisions along both sides of the rib cage. Lift the cut section of the chest wall and remove the heart by cutting the aorta at the base of the chest cavity. Immediately transfer the heart to a weighing boat placed on ice containing cold buffer (4°C). While the heart is in the cold buffer, carefully remove all attached tissue and with extreme care, expose the aorta from connecting tissue. A long piece of aorta is essential for successful operation of the Langendorff heart. Holding the tip of the aorta with two forceps, lift the heart from the cold buffer and place on the aortic perfusion cannula, which should have buffer running through it at a low flow rate. Clamp the aortic stump with a bull dog clamp and tie the the aorta (below its branches) to the apparatus using surgical thread. Increase buffer flow gradually while monitoring flow pressure. If the procedure is successful, the heart begins to beat spontaneously as it warms up, coronary arteries begin to dilate, and buffer flow flushes blood out of the heart. During the first 10 to 15 min, increase buffer flow gradually to reach 60 mm Hg flow pressure (for the guinea pig heart). Next, make a small incision through the left atrium and carefully insert the deflated latex balloon into the left ventricle. Gradually inflate the balloon with saline and monitor ventricular pressure and rate of contraction as an index of heart performance. At an optimum balloon size (0.5 to 0.8 ml for guinea pig heart), ventricular developed pressure and maximal rate of increase in pressure (dP/dt_{max}) reaches a maximum. Overinflating the balloon leads to a decrease in developed pressure. The heart is stimulated with platinum electrodes placed on the surface of the right atrium by gradually increasing the voltage until the heart rate increases to the rate of stimulation. This voltage is identified as the threshold voltage. Stimulate the heart at double its threshold voltage throughout the experiment. If cardiac rhythm is irregular, the rate of stimulation can be altered to attain a regular heart beat. If altering the rate of stimulation does not halt the arrhythmia, stop pacing the heart and restart the stimulation to obtain the new threshold voltage. Buffer flow rate, balloon size, and rate of stimulation can be adjusted to reach optimum conditions and then should be kept constant throughout the experiment. Allow the heart to perform under these optimal conditions for 15 to 30 min to ensure a steady baseline contractility before applying any agents or conditions for studying cardiac response and performance.

3.4. Measurement of Cardiac Performance

Mechanical performance of the heart is monitored by the balloon inserted inside the left ventricle. Altering the balloon size allows the investigator to monitor the relationship between ventricular volume and pressure development by the heart. As the ventricle is comprised of muscle fibers oriented in different directions, the balloon favors the detection of contractility of all ventricular muscle fibers. In addition, a fixed size of the balloon keeps muscle fibers at a constant length throughout the experiment, thus preventing muscle fiber length alterations from interfering in cardiac responses to applied agents and stimuli. Intraventricular pressure developed by the left ventricle is detected by the pressure transducer and the signal is amplified and recorded by the polygraph. Rate of increase in ventricular pressure, denoted as +dP/dt and measured in units of mm Hg/s, is recorded simultaneously by the polygraph via a signal differentiator. Maximal rate of increase in intraventricular pressure during each contraction cycle, denoted as $+dP/dt_{max}$, is commonly used as an index of ventricular contractility. In addition, –dP/dt is used as an index of ventricular muscle relaxation. Intraventricular pressure, +dP/dt, and –dP/dt are sensitive to alterations in cardiac temperature, perfusion pressure, balloon size, and heart rate. Thus, all of these conditions should be kept constant throughout the experiment and in related studies to obtain reliable and consistent results.

4. Potential Problems

This section describes some difficulties one might encounter in preparing a Langendorff heart preparation.

4.1. Inadequate Heparinization

A deep-needle penetration will result in injection of heparin into the gut. This usually results in inadequate heparinization and occlusion of the coronary arteries, with blood clots and appearance of ischemic sections as an outcome. It is best to start a new heart preparation when this occurs.

4.2. Air Bubble Accumulation

Air bubbles may build up in the trap over time and enter the heart. Hence, adequate buffer should be present in the air bubble trap at the start of experiment. Should buffer level drop, momentarily release pressure in the air bubble trap by opening the B1 valve (Figure 2). This will increase the buffer level in the trap.

4.3. Quality of Perfusion Buffer

It is essential to use distilled water and high quality reagents in the buffer. Buffers can be filtered through 0.45-μm pore size cellulose acetate filters before use. Using particle-free buffer ensures a longer period of unaltered heart function. Normally the heart can beat at 30°C for 5 to 6 h without a significant decline in basal contractility. Bacterial growth in the water supply or reagents can also deteriorate heart function due to the release of toxins and proteases from the bacteria. It is essential to wash the apparatus thoroughly with distilled water before and after each experiment.

4.4. Experimental Variations

Minimizing variations in results obtained from different experiments is the key to obtaining reliable data. This can be achieved either by increasing the number of observations or by normalizing data as percentage of control. Moreover, it is recommended that animals within a narrow range of age and weight be selected throughout the study.

References

1. Langendorff, O., *Arch. Gesamte Physiol.*, 61, 291, 1895.
2. Fawzi, A. B. and McNeill, J. H., Effect of neuraminidase treatment on the inotropic response to ouabain, isoproterenol, and calcium in the guinea pig heart, *Eur. J. Pharmacol.*, 112, 295, 1985.
3. Fawzi, A. B. and McNeill, J. H., Effect of lanthanum on the inotropic response of isoproterenol: role of the superficially bound calcium, *Can. J. Physiol. Pharmacol.*, 63, 1106, 1985.
4. Neely, J. R. and Rovetto, M. J., Techniques for perfusing isolated rat hearts, in *Methods in Enzymology*, vol. 39, Hardman, J. G. and O'Malley, B. W., Eds., Academic Press, New York, 1975, 43.
5. Crass III, M. F., McCaskill, E. S., and Shipp, J. C., Effect of pressure development on glucose and palmitate metabolism in perfused heart, *Am. J. Physiol.*, 216, 1569, 1969.

6. Liu, J., Casley, D. J., and Nayler, W. G., Ischemia causes externalization of endothelin-1 binding sites in rat cardiac membranes, *Biochem. Biophys. Res. Commun.*, 164, 1220, 1989.

7. Liu, J., Chen, R., Casley, D. J., and Nayler, W. G., Ischemia and reperfusion increases 125I-labeled endothelin-1 binding in rat cardiac membranes, *Am. J. Physiol.*, 258, H829, 1990.

8. Karwatowska-Porkopczuk, E. and Wennmalm, A., Effects of endothelin on coronary flow, mechanical performance, oxygen uptake, and formation of purines and on outflow of prostacyclin in the isolated rabbit heart, *Circ. Res.*, 66, 46, 1990.

9. Baydoun, A. R., Peers, S. H., Cirino, G., and Woodward, B., Effects of endothelin-1 on the rat isolated heart, *J. Cardiovasc. Pharmacol.*, 13 (Suppl. 5), S193, 1989.

10. Krebs, H. A. and Henseleit, K., *Hoppe-Seylers Z. Physiol. Chem.*, 210, 33, 1932.

Chapter **2**

The Working Rat Heart Preparation

Robert L. Rodgers

Contents

0-8493-3332-6/97/$0.00+$.50
© 1997 by CRC Press, Inc.

1. Introduction

Since the pioneering work of Morgan, Neely, and others in the 1960s,[1,2] the working rat heart preparation has been used widely and very productively for studying the physiology, pathophysiology, biochemistry, and pharmacology of the heart. As the name implies, the principal improvement of this technique over the older Langendorff (retrograde coronary perfusion) method is the ability to perform external hydraulic work. In addition, the direction of fluid flow in the working heart system is a better approximation of physiologic fluid dynamics than is simple back-perfusion of the coronary arteries. The two major applications of this technique are quantification of intact ventricular function and measurements of cardiac fuel metabolism. In addition, the working heart method is a reliable and sensitive indicator of inotropic and chronotropic drug effects on the intact heart. Minor modifications can be conveniently implemented in order to accommodate specific experimental requirements such as the imposition of acute regional or global ischemia[3,4] or the quantification of oxygen consumption and energetic efficiency.[5] Once the basic working rat heart technique is mastered, it can then be easily adapted to hearts of other species such as the guinea pig,[6] or even to smaller rodents such as the hamster or mouse.[7] The purpose of this article is not to provide an exhaustive review of the history or multiple applications and variations of this method. Instead, this discussion is intended to focus on basic details of the methodology itself. Particular emphasis is placed on the more intricate but important aspects of the technique which are not often described thoroughly in research articles, but which could be very practical to investigators who are considering the use of this method for the first time. These include a summary of the basic procedural steps (Section 2), detailed descriptions of the design of the apparatus itself (Section 3), procedures for isolation of the heart and attaching it to the perfusion system (Section 4), a discussion of the types of information which can be obtained using this method (Section 5), and guidelines for recognizing and avoiding potential problems (Sections 6 and 7). Specific applications to the study of basic intact heart mechanical function and of responsiveness to inotropic and chronotropic agents are presented in Sections 3 and 5. The use of the technique for investigations of cardiac metabolism[8,9] is discussed in Chapter 1.

2. Summary of Procedural Steps

Overall, the essential elements in the operational sequence can be summarized as a checklist of four major steps. Detailed descriptions and discussions of the procedure are provided in the subsequent sections.

1. Preparation of the apparatus

Prepare the perfusate either the day before (albumin-containing) or on the day of the experiment (albumin-free). Assemble all components of the perfusion system. Check all connections, calibrate the transducers and other instruments, and fill the apparatus with oxygenating perfusate. Allow the perfusate to reach operating temperature and continue to oxygenate for at least 45 min prior to the isolation and perfusion of the heart.

2. Preparation of the animal

Inject the animal with heparin, prepare the surgical area, and anesthetize the animal if necessary, approximately 10 min before removing the heart. Just prior to heart removal, replace all standing perfusate in the Langendorff perfusion lines and atrial inflow tubing with warm and freshly oxygenated solution.

3. Removal of the heart and attachment to the mounting assembly

Kill the animal according to institutional and Federal guidelines, isolate and trim the heart as quickly as possible, affix the aorta to the aortic cannula, and initiate Langendorff (retrograde) perfusion.

4. Initiation of working heart perfusion and preparation for data acquisition

Insert the intraventricular catheter if required, affix the left atrium to its cannula, attach electrodes for pacing or an electrocardiogram, place the heart in the heart chamber if present, and reroute the perfusate flow from retrograde to the working mode. Check all measurements to be sure that the perfusate flow is uninterrupted and directed appropriately, the cannulas are oriented properly, and that the measurements of pressure, flow, and heart rate are within expected limits. Allow the heart to stabilize 5 to 10 min before pacing (if required) and subsequent data collection.

3. General Description of the Apparatus

3.1. Components of the System

There are essentially three components to the working heart system:

1.   The mounting assembly usually consisting of two cannulas, one for the aorta and the other for the left atrium (Figure 1A).

2.   The left atrial filling system, which commonly incorporates the mechanism for oxygenation of the perfusate, and which is adjustable to establish the level of left atrial filling pressure (Figure 1B); and

3.   The outflow system, providing either fixed or adjustable back-pressure or resistance to the ejection of perfusate from the left ventricle through the aortic remnant and aortic cannula (Figure 1C). Commercial sources for perfusion apparatuses or components include Kontes® (884600), Kent Scientific® (TIS 120140), Hugo Sachs Elektronik® (HSE Type 830), and others. The apparatus illustrated in Figure 1 is based on the Kontes® system as first reported by Morgan and co-workers,[9] with some modification.

3.2.   Open and Closed Designs

Working heart perfusion systems can be categorized as "open" and "closed" (Figure 1). The difference is determined primarily by the type of oxygenator and perfusate employed. Technically, both designs are open to the atmosphere. However, the "closed" system is so designated because the gas is contained within the entire apparatus and its only escape is through a line which can be connected to a KOH or other alkaline trap for accumulation of radioactive CO_2 during metabolism of ^{14}C-containing fuels. If the trap is incorporated, it will then exert an unavoidable ambient back-pressure on the heart in excess of normal atmospheric pressure, which can be severe enough to impede coronary flow. The flow of the gas mixture should be well regulated and kept at a minimum (generating 3 to 7 mm Hg within the system) to avoid significant coronary ischemia. This pressure should be verified with a low-pressure transducer connected to one of the oxygenation lines, and monitored continually in order to ensure steady pressure and thus the absence of any gas leaks in the system.

There are also two basic oxygenator designs (Figure 1B). In the one which is used with the "closed" system, the perfusate usually contains albumin (see below) and coats the walls of the oxygenating vessel in a thin film. The gas flows at a relatively slow rate through the center of the vessel and oxygenates the perfusate by diffusion (Figure 1B, left). "Open" systems usually incorporate a dispersion-type oxygenator, in which the perfusate is vigorously gassed through a fritted disk at the base of the perfusate well (Figure 1B, right). For purposes of discussion, the terms "closed" and "open" systems will henceforth be used to designate oxygenation by diffusion and dispersion, respectively.

3.3. Selection and Preparation of the Perfusate

Of course, any one of several standard balanced salt solutions can be used with this preparation. In practice, the type which seems to have gained the most favor in recent years is some version of Krebs-Henseleit (K-H) solution, varying in only minor respects from one laboratory to another. The formula we use is as follows[10] (concentrations in millimolar): NaCl (120); KCl (5.6); $MgSO_4$ (0.65); NaH_2PO_4 (1.21); $NaHCO_3$ (19 to 25); $CaCl_2$ (1.8 to 2.4). The most common exogenous fuel is glucose, usually between 8 and 12 mM. Of course, any other soluble fuel, such as pyruvate, beta-hydroxybutyrate, or lactate, can be substituted or supplemented at the desired concentrations.[8] When glucose is present, insulin is often added to enhance glucose uptake.[11]

It is convenient to prepare a concentrated buffer stock solution (some warming may or may not be required depending on room temperature) of the following weights (g) for every four liters of volume: NaCl, 561; $CaCl_2$ ($2H_2O$), 28.22 (to yield 2.4 mM); NaH_2PO_4 (H_2O), 13.36; $MgSO_4$ ($7 H_2O$), 13.10; KCl, 33.40. The stock solution should be stored at room temperature. In preparing the final perfusate, appropriate amounts of glucose and sodium bicarbonate are dissolved in deionized water, and then the buffer stock is added in the proportion of 100 ml to every 1900 ml glucose-bicarbonate solution.

The K-H perfusate is gassed with a mixture of 95% O_2, 5% CO_2. When fully saturated, this should yield a pH of close to 7.4 at 37°C. It is recommended that the pH of the gassed perfusate is verified at regular and frequent intervals. The pH can be controlled by varying the amount of sodium bicarbonate (usually between 15 and 25 mM). The required bicarbonate concentration may vary because the CO_2 content of the gas mixture may not be exactly 5%. After the plumbing of the apparatus has been filled, the buffer should be allowed to oxygenate for at least 45 min prior to heart perfusion to ensure complete saturation and the attainment of a stable pH. Just prior to mounting the heart, all standing perfusate should be replaced with warm and fully oxygenated solution, particularly the perfusate in the coronary perfusion line. The required volume of perfusate depends on the design of the apparatus. In the Kontes-type recirculating system, a volume of 100 ml is typical. In any open, nonre-circulating system, the volume contained in the perfusate reservoir feeding the oxygenator can be as much as 8 to 10 liters with suitable vessels, depending on the number of planned perfusions for that day.

The perfusate described above is used without further modification for the open perfusion system. However, the diffusion-type oxygenator of the closed system requires that some albumin be added to the perfusate for two reasons: (1) to allow sheeting of the perfusate over the entire inside surface of the oxygenator, which is necessary for full oxygenation; and (2) to bind to fatty acids which may be included in the perfusate. Simple gassing of fatty acid–albu-min-containing solutions by dispersion results in unmanageable frothing. For fatty acid perfusion, the standard albumin concentration is 3% (3 g/100 ml).

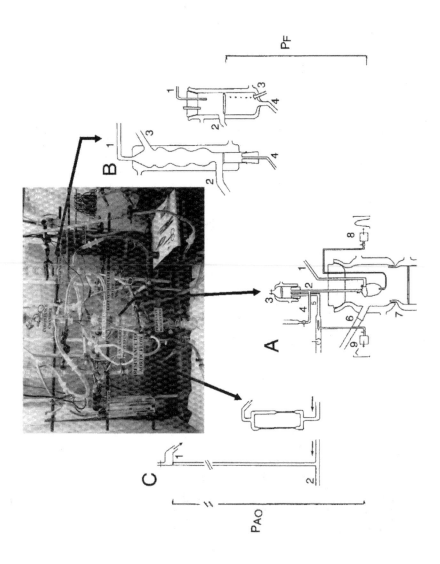

Figure 1

Schematic diagram of the working heart perfusion apparatus. Three main components are highlighted: (**A**) the heart chamber and mounting assembly; (**B**) the inflow (volume loading) and oxygenation system; and (**C**) the outflow (pressure loading) system. The major components of the mounting assembly (**A**) are the inflow (left atrial) cannula (**1**), the outflow (aortic) cannula (**2**), the windkessel compliance chamber (**3**), a sidearm assembly for Langendorff pre-perfusion (**4**), the outflow going to the pressure loading component (**5**), a return conduit (**6**) containing perfusate and oxygen/CO_2 to accommodate the overflow from the oxygenator together with the aortic flow (recirculating design), a perfusate reservoir attached to the bottom of the heart chamber (**7**), and two pressure transducers, one for left ventricular pressure (**8**), and one for aortic pressure (**9**). Two oxygenator designs (**B**) are illustrated, one in which the perfusate coats the inside of the vessel and is oxygenated by diffusion (left), and another in which the perfusate is oxygenated by gas dispersion (right). The height of the perfusate in the oxygenator relative to the heart determines left atrial inflow pressure (**P**F). Both oxygenator designs incorporate perfusate inlets (**1**), perfusate overflows (**2**), gas inlets (**3**), and perfusate outlets to the heart (**4**). In the oxygenator design illustrated, both the perfusate and gas overflows are carried away from the oxygenator in the same tubing. In recirculating designs, the perfusate (oxygenator overflow and aortic flow) is returned from the reservoir to the oxygenator by a peristaltic pump. In nonrecirculating designs (applies only to the dispersion oxygenator), only the overflow is pumped back to a reservoir, while cardiac output is directed to a drain. The pressure loading component (**C**) usually consists of either a column of perfusate of adjustable height (left) or one or more sections of small-diameter tubing imparting adjustable resistances to aortic outflow (right). In the column design, some provision should be made to maintain the desired height (**P**Au) if necessary. This can be done by attaching a low-output rotary pump at the base of the column (**2**), which could be activated to maintain overflow at the top of the column (**1**), should left ventricular contractility become insufficient to maintain a positive aortic flow (such as during recovery from ischemia). If radioactive CO_2 is to be retrieved, the perfusate must not be exposed to air. When the column is used, the overflow could be directed via a large conduit (Tygon® tubing) attached to the overflow line, going from the oxygenator to the heart chamber. If resistances are used instead, they can be housed in a loop going from the aortic outflow line back to the heart chamber. The arrows indicate the direction of perfusate flow. The whole apparatus as shown is based, with some modification, on the Kontes® rat heart perfusion system as reported by Morgan and co-workers (Reference 9). For further details, see text Sections 3.1 and 3.2, and 3.5 to 3.8.

However, if fatty acids are not to be included, then a BSA level of as low as 0.2% is sufficient to ensure full sheeting of the perfusate within the oxygenator.[9] The fatty acid-containing perfusate is prepared by dissolving the albumin in Krebs-Henseleit or other suitable balanced salt solution at about 35 to 38°C while gently stirring. Overheating may cook the BSA and cause it to precipitate out of solution. Simple fraction V BSA is suitable for these applications. It may take 20 or 30 min for the BSA to dissolve. During the final 10 min, an appropriate amount of palmitate or other fatty acid is dissolved in 7 ml of 100% ethanol, and then 10 ml water is added and the mixture is heated to boiling. As soon as the ethanol is boiled off, the fatty acid solution is added quickly to the BSA-buffer solution. The buffer may briefly turn cloudy and then clarify. If it remains cloudy, then the fatty acid did not dissolve, and the buffer should be discarded. The BSA-buffer containing the fatty acid is then dialyzed (MW cutoff of 6000 to 8000, such as Spectra/Por® 132675) overnight at 4°C against 10 X volume of BSA-free Krebs-Henseleit buffer, and used the next day. The perfusate can be stored in the refrigerator, but should not be used any later than 3 days after its preparation.

Thus, the inclusion of fatty acids in the perfusate requires albumin, which in turn necessitates the use of a diffusion-type oxygenator. Whenever ^{14}C-containing fuels are included, a closed system containing an alkaline trap is necessary. If the radioactive fuel is a fatty acid, then the diffusion-type oxygenator must be incorporated into the closed system. However, if all fuels are water-soluble, then either oxygenator design can be employed, with or without an alkaline trap as required. In the closed system, the perfusate is recirculated, but in the open system with a dispersion oxygenator, the perfusate is most often nonrecirculated.

3.4. Temperature Regulation

The means of temperature control is influenced by the system's design. In both systems, perfusate temperature is controlled by jacketed reservoirs and recirculating thermostatic circulation pumps. In the closed system design, the heart must be contained within a jacketed chamber (Figure 1A), and the temperature of the gas surrounding the heart is also controlled by the recirculating water pump. The use of dispersion-type oxygenators in open systems does not necessarily require a jacketed heart chamber. Instead, the entire assembly can be housed in a Plexiglas or wooden box with a Plexiglas door, and the ambient temperature controlled with a thermostat connected to a heat lamp or a similar device. Regardless of the design, the temperature must be regulated as accurately and precisely as possible, because both heart rate and mechanical function are strongly affected by even slight variations in either ambient or perfusate temperature.

3.5. Mounting Assembly and Importance of Cannula Size and Orientation

A typical mounting assembly for a commercially available perfusion apparatus is shown diagrammatically in Figure 1A. Most often, the cannulas are made of stainless steel, although they can be hard plastic or glass. Steel is preferred because it is more rigid than plastic and more durable than glass. The steel should not be cleaned in acid, however, because of the risk of enhanced contamination of the perfusate with metal cations. It would also be helpful if the soldering connections were made with an inert element such as gold. Silver solder can be less durable than gold, and often contains copper, which can be cardiotoxic.

The orientation of the mounting cannulas is of critical importance to the function of the perfused heart. Of course, rat hearts are fairly small, so that minor variations in the angle and position of the filling cannula relative to the aortic cannula can lead to restrictions in either left atrial filling or aortic ejection or both. The problem assumes even greater significance when adapting the method to the perfusion of hearts from smaller rodents such as hamsters, gerbils, or mice.[7] To ensure unencumbered filling, the position of the filling cannula relative to the aortic cannula should be universally and easily adjustable. This can be accomplished by creating a custom-designed assembly. However, in commercially available perfusion apparatuses, the two cannulas in the mounting assembly are generally held parallel to each other at a fixed distance. This arrangement impedes fine adjustments necessary for unrestricted inflow. When encountering atypically low ventricular pressures, one of the first troubleshooting procedures should be a check of cannula positions and patency (see Section 7). When this component of the preparation is functioning properly, full ballooning of the left atrium during diastole will be obvious.

The size of the aortic cannula can also have a profound influence on heart function. The inside diameter of the aorta should be close to the outside diameter of the cannula. If the cannula is too large, then the aorta can be overstretched, leading to partial occlusion of the openings of the coronary arteries secondary to the intrusion of the cannula itself or to edema resulting from the trauma to the aortic tissue. If it is too small, the cannula may contribute inappropriately to the resistance to outflow. In addition, folding of the aortic wall may occur on ligation, promoting leakage and potentially impeding coronary flow. The aortic cannula is usually either flanged at the tip or grooved just proximal to the end, to accommodate the ligature and to prevent the heart from slipping off during perfusion. Either design is acceptable, but a grooved cannula which has been bevelled at a 30 to 45° angle seems to be relatively more amenable to rapid cannula insertion and clamping than the unbevelled, flanged type. Recommended aortic cannula sizes for hearts of different wet weights are given in Table 1.

The size of the atrial inflow cannula is much less critical and less dependent on heart size. Nevertheless, it is important that the lumen of the cannula

TABLE 1
Recommended Cannula Sizes for Rat Hearts of Different Weights[a]

Wet heart weight (g)	Aortic cannula		Left atrial cannula	
	I.D. (in.)	O.D. (in.)	I.D. (in.)	O.D. (in.)
<1.2 g	0.063	0.083	0.071	0.095
1.2 to 2.0 g	0.085	0.109	0.080	0.104

[a] These cannula dimensions and heart weight categories should be viewed as guidelines and not absolute requirements. At least two sets of cannulas should be kept on hand to allow rapid and convenient adjustments for rats of different sizes (see text Section 3.5). Rat hearts weighing more than 2 g may require a third set of larger cannulas. For guinea pig hearts of the same weight, somewhat larger aortic cannulas may be necessary.

be above a minimum diameter to allow unrestricted inflow at the normal operating filling pressures, which are usually between 5 and 25 cm H_2O. It is necessary to establish at the outset that uninterrupted flow rates exceed the maximum expected cardiac output for all anticipated heart sizes, and at all filling pressures and beating frequencies within the usual operating range. Typically, total cardiac output (as the sum of apparent coronary flow and aortic flow rates) is about 30 ml/min per gram wet weight of the whole heart, depending on such factors as the design of the perfusion apparatus (particularly of the outflow system; see Section 3.7), heart size (which can be in excess of 3 g in very large rats), the settings of volume load and pressure load, and beating frequency. Therefore, the velocity of inflow should be sufficient to accommodate extreme peak flow rates of 90 ml/min at beating frequencies which may exceed 300 per minute. Otherwise, Starling curves might be artificially low or displaced to the right, and other indices of function, such as dP/dt, obtained at a fixed filling pressure, might be artificially depressed. Too often, however, the inflow cannulas of commercially available apparatuses are actually larger than they need to be, particularly for 1- to 2-g hearts, requiring excessively large holes in the atrium to accommodate them. Oversized cannulas increase the risk of atrial overdissection with subsequent leakage and electrophysiologic abnormalities, occlusion of the coronary artery upon ligation to the cannula, and difficulties in achieving appropriate geometric orientations. As is true for the aortic cannula, the inflow cannulas can be either flared or grooved. However, bevelling does not seem to have as much of an impact on insertion and ligation of the inflow cannula as it does on the aortic cannula. Recommended inflow cannula sizes are included in Table 1.

3.6. Inflow System and Regulation of Volume Loading

Regardless of the design of the oxygenator (Figure 1B), the volume loading (left atrial filling pressure or P_f), is most commonly regulated by the height of the meniscus relative to the heart. For a variety of valid reasons, the volume load (left atrial filling pressure) should be controlled by gravity-fed constant pressure — and not, for example, by constant flow (as with a peristaltic pump), by flow restriction,[7] or by a pressure head in the oxygenator — regardless of the heart weight or animal species. With gravity-feed atrial filling, variations in heart size are automatically accommodated by appropriate adjustments of the cannula diameters, while diastolic volume is independently determined by the heart itself at a given diastolic filling pressure. The design should allow an adjustable height of 5 to 25 cm, the normal operating range for Frank-Starling curves. The operational constant pressure setting most commonly selected is between 10.0 and 12.5 cm H_2O (13.8 cm H_2O = 10.0 mm Hg = 1.333 kPa). This setting yields left ventricular peak pressures of about 80 to 90% of the peak value on the Frank-Starling curve when the left ventricle ejects into an imposed resistance rather than into a pressure head generated by a standing column of buffer. However, the relationship between left atrial filling pressure and left ventricular developed pressure or cardiac output is influenced substantially by the type of outflow system selected (see Section 3.7 below and Figure 2).

3.7. Outflow System and Regulation of Pressure Loading

Adjustment of the "pressure load," or outflow impedance, against which the left ventricle must eject is an important consideration in the design of isolated working heart systems. Several designs have been implemented with either the open or the closed perfusion system (for an illustration of the "Starling resistor," for example, see Noresson et al.[12] or the HSE catalog). In recent years, one of two designs seems to be preferred by most investigators (Figure 1C): (1) a "column design," consisting of a pressure head created by a standing column of buffer, the meniscus of which is usually between 80 and 120 cm above the heart (Figure 1C, left); and (2) a "resistance design," consisting of one or more sections of small-diameter (PE) tubing or simple syringe needles, usually situated at heart level (Figure 1C, right).

In the column design, the pressure load (P_{Ao}) is simply determined by the height of a standing column of perfusate relative to the heart (Figure 1C, left). The usual operational column height is around 80 to 120 cm, depending on such factors as desired load, strain of rat, animal species, experimental aims, and so forth. Because the height must be kept constant, the column must be distinct from the Langendorff inflow line, unless a recirculation/overflow is built into the Langendorff perfusate reservoir. However, there may be times, such as during ischemia or negatively inotropic drug administration, when the contractility of the heart is insufficient to sustain the desired height of the perfusate within the column. One way to avoid this problem would be to connect a peristaltic pump (drawing from the perfusate reservoir) to the base of the column (#2 in Figure 1C, left). The speed of the pump should be just sufficient to maintain minimal overflow at the top of the column until such time as adequate contractility is restored. Of course, measurements of aortic flow during these periods would be invalid. For metabolic studies involving fuels labeled with ^{14}C, the column must be enclosed within a space continuous with the circulating O_2/CO_2 mixture to prevent the escape of radioactive CO_2 from the perfusate into the surrounding air. Under those conditions, P_{Ao} would be the difference between the column height and the ambient pressure created by the KOH trap at the end of the gas line.

In the multiple resistance design, the plumbing is arranged such that the outflow can be directed quickly and conveniently through any of several tubing sections, which vary in their length or diameter[10] (Figure 1C, right), or through needles of different gages. Each resistance is calibrated by measuring the pressure in the system at several constant flow rates, imposed by a syringe pump stepwise between roughly 5 and 20 cm^3 (ml) per minute, and then determining the slope of the resulting pressure-flow plot. For rat hearts weighing between 1.0 to 2.0 g, a resistance of around 1.0 $kPa/cm^3/min$ should yield peak left ventricular pressure values of approximately 16 kPa (120 mm Hg). However, resistance settings should be adjusted to allow for large differences in heart size. For example, rat hearts exceeding 2 g would be expected to generate significantly greater stroke volumes than 1-g hearts. Since $P = QR$, the resistance should be adjusted empirically to yield left ventricular peak pressures which are within a certain acceptable operating range in the face of significant differences in cardiac output (Q). In other words, if larger hearts are exposed to resistances designed for significantly smaller hearts, the resulting peak left ventricular pressures will be inappropriately high (perhaps 140 to 150 mm Hg instead of the more reasonable 120). Thus, cardiac function analyses should be carried out on hearts of approximately equal mass, or appropriate controls should be included.[10] To generate pump function curves for hearts weighing approximately 1 to 1.5 g, the multiple resistance settings should lie between 0.5 and 2.0 $kPa/cm^3/min$. Lower resistances can be imposed for short periods. However, anything lower than about 0.6 (somewhat higher for concentrically hypertrophic hearts from hypertensive rats) may fall below the resistance of the coronary vascular bed, imposing ischemic conditions.

The genetic strain of the animal is another important factor when establishing the level of loading conditions. Normotensive rats, such as the Sprague-Dawley or Wistar, have lower coronary resistance than either the moderately hypertensive Wistar-Kyoto or the fully hypertensive spontaneously hypertensive rat (SHR) strain. The SHR uniformly requires relatively higher columns or resistances to maintain stable function.

A suitable compliance ("windkessel") chamber should also be included in the design. Usually, this consists of a simple bubble trap inserted into the aortic outflow line (Figure 1A). The volume of air in the trap should be adjustable, to regulate the magnitude of aortic pulse pressure (systolic – diastolic). The greater the volume, the narrower the pulse pressure. A volume between 3 and 5 ml is typical, yielding physiologically representative aortic pulse pressures of around 30 to 40 mm Hg. The use of flexible latex tubing in the aortic outflow circuit will add to the compliance, but will also favor the escape of oxygen from the perfusate by diffusion, and may artifactually distort the shape of the aortic pressure wave.

3.8.   Advantages and Disadvantages of Different Components and System Designs

Each system — open and closed — has its own set of strengths and weaknesses. The major advantages of the open system without albumin and with dispersion oxygenation are that the perfusate is more conveniently prepared and perfusate oxygenation seems to be closer to full saturation, allowing the imposition of relatively greater workloads without compromising mechanical function. However, without fatty acids in the perfusate, metabolic support of contraction is more dependent on endogenous triglycerides. Even with glucose and insulin in the medium, stable function begins to decline as the triglycerides are depleted, usually within 1 to 2 hours, depending on the workload and beating frequency. The duration of stable function seems to be prolonged when high concentrations of pyruvate (e.g., 5 mM) are supplied instead of glucose, even though these levels of pyruvate are sufficient to completely shut down fatty acid oxidation.

The closed system is more convenient, simpler in its design and maintenance, and requires less perfusate for the support of contraction. Maintenance of stable function in the closed system with the thin-film oxygenator, however, seems to require adjustments to somewhat lower workloads, with correspondingly decreased values of left ventricular peak pressure and dP/dt. This may be a consequence of relatively restricted saturation of the perfusate with oxygen by diffusion-type oxygenators. Very often in the closed system the hearts are allowed to beat spontaneously rather than paced, and values for work are expressed as rate–pressure product (which is assumed to be directly and linearly proportional to oxygen consumption) rather than Joules or Watts at a fixed beating frequency (see Section 5.6). In the closed system, the availablility of exogenous fatty acids and the imposition of lower workloads are sufficient to support stable mechanical function for at least 2 h, as long as the pacing frequency is not excessively high (greater than 300 per minute). Containment of oxygen can be improved by using low-diffusion tubing such as Pharmed®. The oxygen-carrying capacity of the perfusate can be enhanced with the addition of packed red cells or artificial hemoglobin[13,14] or by perfusing with whole blood from donor animals. These modifications improve the physiologic integrity of the method, but also impose significantly greater expense and technical complexity, and are thus beyond the scope of this discussion. As a general rule, the open system is satisfactory for the short-term analysis of mechanical function and pharmacological responsiveness (see Sections 5.1 and 5.4), while the closed system is more appropriate for the study of cardiac metabolism (see Chapter 2 of Book 3).

Either of the pressure loading designs can be used with the open or closed systems, and each has its own set of advantages and disadvantages. It must be borne in mind that the coronary vasculature is a parallel component of the total resistance to aortic outflow, regardless of which type of pressure load is selected. Thus, one advantage of the buffer column is that it provides a constant minimum coronary perfusion pressure (diastolic aortic pressure), regardless of the contractile state of the left ventricle or heart size. In that regard, the design is reminiscent of a constant-pressure Langendorff system. This feature may be useful, for example, when testing the effects of negatively inotropic drugs and toxins, or in ischemia studies to promote recovery from the ischemic episode. Also, the column design yields higher values for aortic flow and greater (more physiologically representative) ratios of aortic-to-coronary flow rates than does the resistance design. However, the constant high pressure on the aortic valve imposed by the column seems to promote leakage and back-flow, leading to overfilling of the left ventricle during diastole. This in turn displaces the Starling curve far to the left — so that the rising phase of the curve is abnormally steep — and upward at the lower filling pressures (Figure 2). Therefore, in that respect the buffer column is relatively nonphysiologic, and not particularly suitable for studies of ventricular function.

The "resistance" design is hemodynamically more representative, in that the level of mean aortic pressure, and thus coronary perfusion pressure, is a function of the inotropic state of the left ventricle. With this design, backflow or regurgitation through the aortic valve does not seem to be as much of a problem, so that the Starling curve is displaced more to the right and its shape is more typical of curves obtained *in vivo* (Figure 2). The resistance design is therefore more appropriate for studies of ventricular function, as long as provisions are made for large differences in heart mass, as discussed above. However, it may be less suitable for studies of acute ischemia. When a fixed resistance rather than a buffer column is used, any acute cardiodepressant intervention (such as very low filling pressure, hypoxia, ischemia, drugs and toxins, metabolic fuel depletion, electrolyte imbalances, etc.) which decreases the contractile state has the potential of initiating and accelerating a downward spiral of diminishing coronary perfusion pressure (mean aortic pressure minus left ventricular pressure), coronary flow, and left ventricular function. Compared to the buffer column design, the resistance design markedly decreases the duration of ischemia from which the ventricle can mechanically recover. Incidentally, the guinea pig heart requires a lower pressure load than the rat heart does — typically on the order of 40 to 60 cm H_2O (standing buffer column) or 0.5 to 0.6 $kPa/cm^3/min$ (resistance design) — because both its coronary vascular resistance and its basal left ventricular inotropic state are lower than those of the rat heart[6,15-17] (see Section 5.4 and Figure 3).

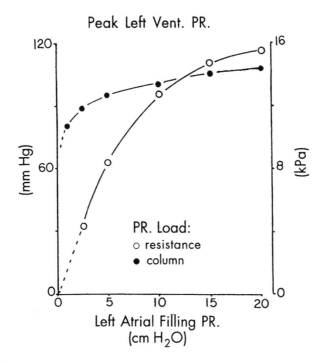

Figure 2

Influences of the pressure loading design on the shape of cardiac function curves. In the figure above, two Frank-Starling curves of a single working rat heart are represented as maximum left ventricular pressure at various volume loads (left atrial filling pressures). The two curves were generated by imposing pressure loads of different design. One (●) consisted of a buffer column 120 cm above the heart, and the other (○) a length (determined empirically) of PE 90 tubing to yield a resistance of 1.0 kPa/cm^3 × min^{-1} (see text Section 3.7 and 3.8). The heart was artificially paced at 275 beats per minute. Note that the column design results in a curve which is relatively flat and shifted to the left. This effect is probably the result of elevated left ventricular diastolic volumes at the lower filling pressures, secondary to semilunar regurgitation or perfusate leakage via other routes. The shape of the curve generated with the resistance design is a better approximation of the Frank-Starling relationship obtained *in vivo*. Data are unpublished.

4.   Isolation of the Heart

4.1.   Preparation of the Animal and Removal of the Heart

Along with the purity of the water, the speed of isolation of the heart is probably the most critical aspect of the entire procedure. The most important considerations for animal preparation and heart removal are rapidity of dissection and avoidance of blood coagulation in the coronary vasculature and ventricular chambers during the isolation procedure. Accordingly, the animal should be injected with heparin (at least 1000 u/kg) intraperitoneally about 10 to 15 min before heart removal. The animal should be rapidly decapitated with or without prior anesthetization with ether, halothane, or other suitable anesthetic, in compliance with institutional and Federal guidelines for animal care and use (check the current AVMA Panel on Euthanasia recommendations). Of course, if anesthetics are to be used, then appropriate control groups designed to isolate the effects of the anesthetic should be included. The chest should be opened rapidly with large surgical scissors, and the heart quickly excised and placed in a dish containing the perfusate at a depth of about 2 cm. Some investigators prefer to chill the dissection perfusate in ice, to accelerate arrest. However, we have done it both ways, and found that maintaining the solution at room temperature does not markedly affect arrest time. In addition, chilling the heart seems to delay the resumption of stable function (i.e., rewarming) once perfusion is initiated, increasing the required stabilization period. As long as the dissection and mounting time is sufficiently brief, neither the level nor the total duration of stable function during perfusion seems to be significantly influenced by the temperature of the heart during trimming and dissection. We have found that trimming and mounting is expedited by using curved forceps and small surgical scissors. During heart excision, care must be taken to leave enough of an aortic remnant for ease of cannulation and to minimize the risk of intrusion by the mounting cannula on the semilunar valve. The aorta should be cut just proximal to the base of the innominate artery. This will provide approximately 5 to 7 mm of aortic remnant to work with, which should leave plenty of room for clamping (with a small "bulldog" or serrefine clamp such as Roboz® RS 7440 or RS 5457) and subsequent ligation of the aorta onto the cannula.

4.2. Attachment of the Heart to the Mounting Assembly

Once the heart — together with any attached lung, thymus, and pericardial tissue — is removed, it must be trimmed and mounted as quickly as possible, preferably within 30 s, but certainly no longer than 60 s. It is very important, just before the animal is killed, to run sufficient perfusate through the aortic perfusion line such that the standing perfusate is replaced by warm, freshly oxygenated solution. Otherwise, the heart may be exposed to hypothermic and hypoxic conditions during the early phases of Langendorff perfusion. It is also important to remove residual thymus and lung prior to mounting. If they are not removed, then the added weight will stretch the aorta, promoting edema and thereafter compromising coronary flow and ventricular function. In addition, it is very useful to separate the aorta from the pulmonary artery with a careful snip using the small dissecting scissors. This will allow the aorta to hang straight down from the cannula, relieving the geometric constraint imposed by the arch of the aorta, thereby minimizing restrictions to aortic outflow and decreasing the risk of edema formation. The cut should be made such that, if a vessel is nicked, it is the pulmonary artery. A small incision must be made in that vessel anyway, to ensure uninterrupted coronary flow after the left atrium is fixed to its cannula, because the pulmonary artery is often coligated with the left atrium to the inflow cannula. If necessary, the pericardium can be trimmed after the heart is attached to the aortic cannula, during retrograde perfusion. The aortic remnant is first clamped onto the cannula and the heart oriented so that the left atrium is facing forward (toward the investigator) and somewhat to the right, and the pulmonary artery is clearly visible. Coronary perfusion should be initiated here, and the aortic remnant tied to the cannula underneath the clamp and above the flange or into the groove. For consistency of attachment and ease of ligation, 3-0 surgical silk (Ethicon®) is recommended.

Once the aorta is ligated to its cannula and retrograde perfusion is initiated, the preparation is essentially a Langendorff heart. If left ventricular pressure of the working heart is to be monitored, then the next step is to insert a pressure probe into the left ventricle (see Section 5.2). After the pressure probe is inserted into the left ventricle, then the inflow cannula is ligated to the left atrium. It may be necessary at this point to implement additional fine dissection of the tissue around the atrium in order to optimize the size and location of the opening. Ideally, the atrium should be trimmed such that the openings of the remnants of the pulmonary veins are just slightly expanded. This can be achieved consistently with practice. As discussed above (Section 3.5), it is important to avoid creating a hole which is too large. Overdissection may make it very difficult to avoid ligating the coronary artery, which lies just below the junction of the left and right atria. It may also impede full filling and expansion of the left atrium, potentially compromising performance. After ligation of the left atrium to its cannula, it is necessary to check the pulmonary artery to make sure that drainage through this vessel is unimpeded. Pulmonary arterial outflow largely represents a mixture of coronary flow from the coronary sinus, combined with any leakage from the left to the right atrium and the right ventricle. Thus, to avoid compromising coronary flow, it is critical that pulmonary arterial flow is unrestricted. If a nick had not been effectively placed in the pulmonary artery during the trimming procedure, then subsequent coligation with the left atrium might result in an obvious distention of the vessel due to occlusion. Should that occur, then a small cut should be quickly placed in the artery at this time. Completeness of left atrial filling should be verified by briefly opening the inflow line and observing the dilation of the atrium. Any leaks around the atria should be corrected here.

As soon as the left atrium is fixed in place, the system is switched over from the Langendorff to the working mode. The first step is to open the inflow tubing from the oxygenator to the left atrium. Then, aortic outflow is quickly rerouted toward either the free-standing buffer column or the resistance assembly (cutting off the Langendorff perfusion vessel). In either the open or closed system, the level of the perfusate in the oxygenator is usually maintained by an overflow regulated by a rotary pump. In our laboratory, left atrial filling pressure in the open system is maintained with a glass float valve situated within a relatively shallow, wide-mouthed dispersion-type oxygenator (of the type illustrated on the right in Figure 1B), rather than by pump-generated overflow. The valve is gravity-fed by a larger primary vessel, also containing gassed perfusate, placed above the oxygenator.

Once the conversion from Langendorff to working perfusion is effected, then stable pressures and spontaneous frequencies should be attained within 5 to 8 min. A triphasic pattern is often observed, consisting of a short hyperactive phase due mainly to endogenous catecholamine release, leading to a brief period of hypofunction, which then should be followed by stable mechanical and electrical activity.

4.3. Pacing and Obtaining an Electrocardiogram

As long as the temperature of the perfusate is well regulated at 37°C, the apparatus is clean, the heart is mounted quickly and properly, and the water used to make the perfusate is very pure, then the spontaneous beating frequency should be stable and fairly consistent between preparations (usually within 250 and 300 beats per minute). However, even slight variations in frequency exert well-known indirect effects on mechanical function. If any element of mechanical activity — such as dP/dt, peak pressure, time to peak pressure, and so forth (see Section 5.4) — is to be quantified and compared with other hearts in different experimental groups, or if inotropic effects of drugs are to be characterized, then no variability of beating frequency is acceptable, and artificial pacing is mandatory. Fortunately, pacing these hearts is easy, whether an open or closed system is used. Suitable electrodes are available commercially, but they can also be conveniently fashioned in the laboratory from two insulated copper wires. Each insulated wire can be soldered to smaller guage wire electrodes made of partially or completely inert metal such as platinum, gold, or stainless steel. The ends of the small wires are bent into a small loop, separated from each other by a distance of about 2 mm, fixed in a suitable clamp or adjustable holder, and placed on the surface of either the left or the right atrium. If the heart is enclosed in a chamber, then each insulated wire is connected to an alligator clamp, one of which is fixed to the inflow cannula and the other to the outflow cannula (Figure 1). The other ends of the copper wires are connected to the + and − poles of the stimulator (such as a GRASS SD 9 or equivalent), which is normally set at a square wave pulse of about 5 msec duration. The required voltage may vary somewhat, but 2 to 4 V is usually sufficient. The voltage should be dialled up until triggered beating is evident from the tachograph tracing, then increased further about 10%.

Consistent pacing can be a problem under certain experimental conditions. For example, atrial pacing of ventricular beating becomes ineffective when atrioventricular blockade is induced by administered drugs or toxins. At times, it may be desirable to separate the negative inotropic effects from the negative chronotropic and dromotropic effects of agents such as acetylcholine. The confounding effects of decreased heart rate and A-V blockade can be overridden by dual pacing. Two separate bipolar electrodes, one on the atrium and the other on the ventricular apex, are connected to a stimulator which has at least two output channels and a delay capability. The delay between the first (atrial) pulse and the second (ventricular) pulse is set at about 20 to 30 milliseconds, but should be determined empirically by each investigator, using the PR interval of the electrocardiogram as a guide. This pacing procedure effectively preserves coordinated and constant atrioventricular contractions during complete A-V block.

Obtaining an electrocardiographic tracing is quite straightforward with the working heart technique. In either the open or closed system, one convenient method is to insert three platinum needle electrodes (such as those provided by GRASS® instruments), one in each atrium and the third in the apex of the ventricles. The wires are connected to a manifold, the cable of which is connected to a suitable coupler in the recording device.[18] The ventricular apex needle is connected to the ground pole, and a standard lead II is used. Of course, if a heart chamber is present, then some accommodation must be provided for the wires to traverse the chamber. This can be done by threading the wires through a hole drilled in the Teflon plug or stopper containing the cannulae, and sealing the opening each time with petroleum jelly or stopcock grease.

5. Data Acquisition

5.1. Quantification of Heart Function

Regardless of the specific aims of any individual study involving the working heart preparation, they almost always require some measurement of basic cardiac function. In most cases, pressure and flow transducers coupled to a chart recorder are all that is necessary. Indeed, very accurate flow measurements can be obtained using ordinary volumetric procedures, if access to outflow is not restricted. Quantification of function can be as simple as peak left ventricular pressure development or as complex as systolic wall stress or pressure-volume loop determinations. For most applications, however, a sufficiently detailed profile of left ventricular function can be easily generated from a relatively few direct and derived measurements. An adequate set of direct measurements should include left ventricular and aortic pressure waveforms, heart rate, and aortic and coronary flow rates. Aortic pressure alone is not a particularly valid index of ventricular function, but it is a useful indirect measurement, and it provides clear and immediate verification that the aortic semilunar valve is intact. Indices of performance derived from these measurements include cardiac output, hydraulic work, hydraulic power, and left ventricular maximum positive and negative dP/dt (see Section 5.5). Performance indices requiring accurate and dynamic determinations of intraventricular volume[19] are much more difficult to obtain with this preparation and are beyond the scope of this discussion.

5.2.   Pressure Measurements

Recordings of intraventricular, aortic, or other pressures (see Figure 1A) are usually accomplished with a thin, fluid-filled catheter, usually made from PE tubing, connected to a suitable pressure transducer (such as Gould®, Viggo-Spectramed®, and others), but solid pressure probes can also be used. Solid catheters such as Millar® are more expensive, but their signals are not subject to dampening by increases in catheter length or decreases in diameter, and are less likely to be influenced by vibration. Obtaining ventricular pressure using an intraventricular balloon catheter requires retrograde coronary perfusion with or without artificial valves, and as such is outside the limits of this discussion. When fluid-filled probes are used, great care must be taken to ensure that the entire line, from the tip of the probe to the interior of the transducer, is free of air bubbles. Also, the catheter tubing should be no smaller than PE 190, and its length should be kept at the minimum imposed by geometric con-straints. Catheters which are too long or narrow, too compliant, or which contain even very small air bubbles, can have a significant dampening effect on the signal. The undampened frequency response of the transducer should be at least 1 kHz (check with the manufacturer for specifications).

The placement of the probes also markedly influences the shape and magnitude of the signal. For aortic pressure determinations, the closer the tip of the catheter is placed to the aortic semilunar valve, the more accurate the reading will be. In practice, the tip of the aortic pressure probe should be placed within the aortic outflow tubing and directed upstream with the tip positioned as close as practical to the aortic cannula. Simple connection with a sidearm or Y fitting will yield dampened signals and artificially low mean pressure readings. Placement of the left ventricular pressure probe is easier to do when using the open perfusion system and the heart is not encased in a chamber. In the presence of a heart chamber, the catheter can be threaded through the Teflon plug or stopper in a manner analogous to that which was described above for electrodes (Section 4.3). Threading the catheter down via the aortic outflow conduit through the semilunar valve (as typified by the HSE apparatus, for example) is a less desirable approach because of the risk of inducing aortic incompetency. One good way to ensure that a fluid-filled catheter will be placed properly inside the left ventricle is to insert it downward through the left atrium. Approximately 5 cm of PE 190 tubing is heat-flared at one end and bevelled to a point on the other, and marked with a felt-tipped pen about 8 mm from the flared end. The bevelled end is then inserted downward through the left atrium into the left ventricle and through the apex, and drawn out until the mark is exposed, leaving the flared end inside the chamber. The tubing can then be cut to any desired length to facilitate con-nection with the second length of tubing going through the plug to the transducer. For both the aortic and ventricular pressure measurements, the transducers should be positioned at heart level (see Figure 1A).

5.3. Flow Measurements

Cardiac output as the sum of aortic and pulmonary arterial flow rates can be measured intermittently, by volumetric or gravimetric methods, or continually with the use of flowmeters connected to in-line flow probes. As discussed above (Section 3.8), it should be borne in mind that pulmonary arterial outflow is usually an overestimate of coronary flow in this preparation, mainly because of leakage from the left atrium to the right side of the heart. However, substantial acute changes in coronary flow caused, for example, by vasoactive agents, can be reliably detected with the working heart preparation. More subtle acute effects, or consequences of chronic interventions *in vivo* such as hypertension or chronic drug treatment, on coronary flow or resistance might be more reliably detected using a Langendorff system.

The method of obtaining flow rates is dependent to some extent on whether the system design includes a closed heart chamber without an accessible drainage port at the bottom. The absence of a heart chamber of course provides more options. The most direct and inexpensive approach is collection, at regular and frequent intervals, of the effluent from the aortic and pulmonary arterial outflows into small graduated cylinders or modified glass pipettes connected to drainage tubing which can be clamped. Pulmonary arterial outflow can be collected as it runs off the apex of the heart, or the artery can be cannulated with a short (3 to 4 cm) length of PE tubing of appropriate diameter. For rat hearts of 1 to 2 g, PE 260 tubing is suitable. The tubing should be cut at an angle on one end, and the cut end slightly heat-flared to facilitate insertion and ligation. The required time for the collection of a predetermined volume is simply determined with a stopwatch. This method is somewhat inconvenient but accurate. An obvious disadvantage, however, is that it is also intermittent, so that subtle and rapid changes in flow rates might be missed. A somewhat more convenient modification of this procedure is the insertion of pressure probes, connected to pressure transducers, inside the drainage tubing below the glass pipette or other narrow collection vessel.[12,20] The tubing is intermittently clamped below the probe, and the linear rise in pressure with time during filling of the collection vessel is recorded. The resulting slope is directly proportional to the flow rate. This approach is also accurate but intermittent. The use of in-line flow probes and flowmeters provides uninterrupted recordings of flow rates, but is less accurate and markedly more expensive. However, they may be the only practical approach to the quantification of aortic and coronary flow rates when access to the heart is restricted by a closed heart chamber. One probe is placed in the left atrial inflow line, and the other in the aortic outflow tubing. The first is an estimate of cardiac output, and the difference between the first and second measurements is an estimate of coronary flow.

5.4. Quantification of Responses to Chronotropic and Inotropic Agents

The perfused working rat and guinea-pig hearts are excellent preparations for studying the responsiveness of cardiac tissue to both chronotropic and inotropic agents (Figure 3). Reproducible cumulative dose-response curves can be obtained using either the nonrecirculating or the recirculating perfusion designs. In the open system, the drugs are added directly to the perfusate, in both the filling reservoir and in any additional reservoirs, from individual concentrated stock dilutions[16,17] corresponding to each dose. All reservoirs should be graduated or marked for the range of perfusate volumes to facilitate the determination of administration volumes from the stock dilutions. Each stock dilution is prepared with appropriate allowances made for the contribution of previous additions. After adding each dose, the connecting tubing should be rapidly drained (through three-way connectors or similar components placed in the connecting lines in anticipation of this application) to minimize dilution errors. When closed systems are employed, the drug stock dilutions can be injected directly into a latex section of a perfusate line. The constant perfusate volume and recirculation greatly simplifies the procedure. Chronotropic effects are obtained using spontaneously beating hearts, while inotropic responses must be obtained from hearts which are electrically paced, particularly if the agent of interest exhibits both inotropic and chronotropic properties. Normally, inotropic effects are quantified in terms of changes in left ventricular positive dP/dt (maximum rate of increase in left ventricular pressure during isovolumic systole), a derived measurement often used as an index of ventricular muscle contractility in these preparations (see Section 5.5 below). Indices of agonist potency (pD_2 as the negative log of the EC_{50}) obtained with the working heart preparation are reliable, precise, and reproducible (Figure 3).

5.5. Data Analysis

A variety of options are open to the investigator with regard to data acquisition and manipulation. For most applications, analog chart recorders (such as the Grass® polygraph, Narco® physiograph, Gould® recording systems, and so forth) with suitable preamplifiers are sufficient for reasonably accurate and precise quantification of left ventricular and aortic pressures, aortic and coronary flow rates, and derived indices such as dP/dt and dQ/dt (flow velocities). Digital recordings can be obtained with more recently available preprogrammed analog-to-digital data acquisition systems such as MacLab®, Po-Ne-Mah®, and others. More sophisticated software packages such as Asyst® allow greater flexibility, but require rather advanced programming skills. An example

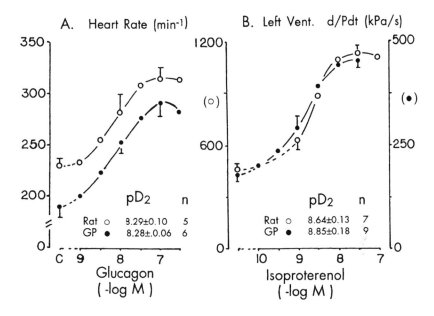

Figure 3
Illustrations of the use of the isolated working heart technique for the analysis of chronotropic (**A**) and inotropic (**B**) actions of drugs and hormones on rat and guinea pig hearts. Chronotropic effects of glucagon (**A**) were obtained from spontaneously beating hearts, while inotropic responses to isoproterenol (**B**) were generated from hearts which were artificially paced at 300 to 320 beats per minute. The nonrecirculating perfusate was Krebs-Henseleit solution (rat) or Chenoweth-Koelle solution (guinea pig) without albumin. Cumulative concentrations were achieved in a nonrecirculating open system by incorporating two oxygenators, a smaller one which determined left atrial perfusion pressure, fed by a larger one which served as reservoir. The agents were added to both vessels from a concentrated stock solution to achieve the desired final concentrations, taking into consideration the contributions of previous additions. Provisions were made to quickly flush out the perfusate in connecting tubing with each administration. In closed recirculating designs, cumulative drug administration would be a much more straightforward process (see text Section 5.4). Note that the basal contraction frequency (**A**) and contractility (**B**) of guinea pig hearts were lower than those of the rat, but that the potencies (pD_2 values) for either glucagon or isoproterenol were not different between species. Data are from References 16 and 17. Inotropic effects of isoproterenol on the rat heart are unpublished.

of digital left ventricular waveform recordings using Asyst® software,[21-23] including illustrations of specific measurements and performance indices, is depicted in Figure 4. The major advantage of digital processing is that, with sufficient resolution, it is much more powerful than analog recording. For example, digital recording greatly facilitates the quantification of time and area intervals which are necessary for detailed determinations of contraction and relaxation parameters.[21,23] The choice of analog or digital data acquisition will, obviously, be influenced by the aims of the study and the degree of detail desired.

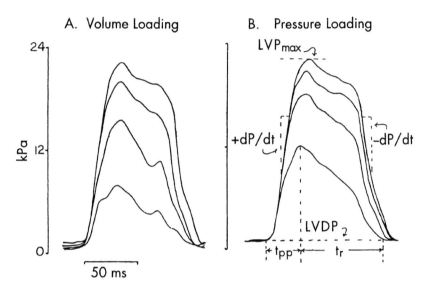

Figure 4

Illustration of the application of digital waveform analysis to the characterization of left ventricular function in the isolated working heart preparation. Left ventricular function of a single heart is expressed two ways: **(A)** by varying volume loading at a fixed pressure load (the typical Frank-Starling relationship); and **(B)** by varying pressure loading at a fixed volume load (used in "pump function" analysis). In A, the four volume loads (left atrial filling pressures) were 5, 10, 15, and 20 cm H_2O (see text Section 3.6), and the pressure load was 1.54 kPa/cm^3 × min^{-1}. In **B**, the four pressure loads (resistances to left ventricular ejection) were 0.19, 0.41, 1.54, and 3.13 kPa/cm^3 × min^{-1} (see text Section 3.7), and the volume load (left atrial filling pressure) was held constant at 15 cm H_2O. The heart was paced at 300 per minute. Analog signals were digitalized and stored on a diskette and regenerated with ASYST® software and an IBM computer with an HP7470® plotter (the plotter output was highlighted for clarity). The A/D conversion board (Data Translation Inc.®) provided for a maximum resolution of 10 microseconds. Note that incremental changes in pressure load **(B)** influence systolic pressure development in a manner which is similar to that of volume loading **(A)**, but without appreciably affecting diastolic pressure (and presumably diastolic volume). The two approaches to the characterization of intact ventricular function as illustrated in **A** and **B** are distantly analogous to pre- and afterloading of ventricular muscle preparations (see Chapter 3 and Reference 21). Among the various measurements which can be accurately determined from these digital waveforms are peak left ventricular systolic pressure (LVP$_{max}$), left ventricular diastolic pressure (LVDP), maximum rates of left ventricular rise and fall (LV + and – dP/dt), time from end-diastole to Pmax (t$_{pp}$), and time from P$_{max}$ to the end of the pressure wave (t$_r$). For an example of a continuous digital output of both P$_{LV}$ and LV dP/dt, see Reference 21. Digitalization markedly expands the power of waveform analysis, and increases the convenience of recording while eliminating distortions due pen inertia or mechanical chart advancement (unpublished data; for more details, see text Section 5.5 and References 21–23).

5.6.   Calculations and Conversions

In the interest of convenience, a list of common conversions, calculations, and derivations is provided below. Of course, units of pressure, flow, and work can be expressed in a variety of ways. The values below are given in cgs units.

Pressure:

$$1 \text{ mm Hg} = 1.38 \text{ cm H}_2\text{O}$$
$$150 \text{ mm Hg} = 20 \text{ kPa}.$$
$$1 \text{ kPa} = 10^4 \text{ dynes/cm}^2 = 10^4 \text{ ergs/cm}^3 = 1 \text{ mJ/cm}^3$$

Flow:

$$60 \text{ ml/min} = 1 \text{ cm}^3/\text{s}$$

Power:

$$1 \text{ mW} = 1 \text{ mJ/s}$$

Work:

$$1 \text{ mJ} = 1 \text{ mW} \times \text{s}$$

Left ventricular pulse pressure (kPa) = peak left ventricular systolic pressure (kPa) – left ventricular end-diastolic pressure (kPa).

Cardiac output (cm^3/s/g) = [aortic flow rate (cm^3/s) + coronary flow rate (cm^3/s)]/wet or dry heart weight (g).

Stroke volume (cm^3/beat per gram) = cardiac output (cm^3/s/g)/heart rate (beats/sec).

Hydraulic power (mW/g) = left ventricular pulse pressure (kPa) × cardiac output (cm^3/s/g)

Stroke work (mJ per beat per gram) = hydraulic power (mW/g)/heart rate (beats per sec) = left ventricular pulse pressure (kPa) × stroke volume (cm^3/beat per gram)

6. Cleaning and Maintaining the Apparatus

For optimum performance, it is critical that both the apparatus and the water used to prepare the perfusate are as clean as possible. Perhaps the most common causes of problems with this technique are impurities in the water and on the surfaces which come in contact with the perfusate. As a general rule, diligent cleaning and frequent replacement of tubing will keep these problems to a minimum.

The procedure for cleaning the apparatus depends somewhat on the design. Typically, open (nonrecirculating) systems with dispersion oxygenators are relatively complex, with a significantly greater number of components and tubing connections. For practical reasons, it is desirable to clean the open system without completely disassembling it. This can be done by copious rinsing of the entire system, first with acidified tap water and then with deionized water, making sure that the inside surfaces of all components come in contact with the rinsing solution. The fittings are then disconnected and the apparatus is allowed to air-dry overnight. All tubing which comes in contact with the perfusate should be replaced regularly, at least once every 2 or 3 weeks. At that time, the glassware should be acid-cleaned as described below. Closed systems (such as the Kontes® apparatus) often are relatively simple in design, and in any case must be disassembled and cleaned daily. The tubing should be rinsed liberally with warm tap water followed by a thorough rinse with deionized water. The tubing should not be cleaned with detergent or chemical disinfectants. All inside surfaces of tubing and connections should be inspected to ensure that they have been rinsed free of albumin deposits. The glassware, particularly the oxygenator and the lower buffer reservoir, must be dipped overnight in concentrated sulfuric acid containing the oxidizing agent ammonium persulfate (approximately 0.5 g/l). Acid-cleaning is necessary to ensure complete coating of the perfusate over the entire inside surface of the oxygenator, and thus maximum possible oxygenation of the perfusate. As stated above, contact with acid of all metal parts must be avoided.

For water purification, a multiple-cartridge deionizing system is recommended. A purity of 16 to 18 MΩ is desirable. An endotoxin removal cartridge is mandatory. The water should be tested weekly for endotoxin contamination. Any detectable trace of endotoxin is cause for alarm. The perfused heart is so sensitive to endotoxin contamination that it can almost be considered a bioassay for it. If highly purified, endotoxin-free water is not available, then this method should not even be considered.

7. Troubleshooting

The following is a selected list of the most commonly encountered problems and some of their more likely sources. Note that either impure water or inadequate cleaning of the apparatus or both are frequent causes.

Observation	Possible causes
Low left ventricular pressure	Impure water
	Improperly cleaned or contaminated tubing, glassware, or fittings
	Inadequate perfusate oxidation; poor gas dispersion or incomplete coating of perfusate on walls of oxygenator
	Resistance or buffer column too low
	Perfusate leak somewhere in the inflow or outflow line

Observation	Possible causes
	Leak in aorta (inadvertently nicked, etc)
	Leak in left atrium, intraventricular catheter, or pressure transducer
	Gas leak in closed system
	Gas pressure too high in closed system
	Temperature too low for the pacing frequency
	Langendorff perfusion line left open
	Perfusate improperly routed; stopcocks improperly set
	Insufficient metabolic fuel or $CaCl_2$, improper pH, or other errors in perfusate preparation
	Improper placement of the pressure probe
	Occlusion or bubble in the fluid-filled catheter probe or transducer
	Misalignment or poor positioning of the left atrial inflow cannula
	Occlusion of the left atrial inflow line
	Oxygenator placed too low relative to the heart
	Oxygenator being drained by cardiac output (i.e., cardiac output exceeding replenishment of perfusate in oxygenator with rotary pump)
	Spontaneous or pacing frequency excessively high
High left ventricular pressure	Errors in perfusate preparation
	Improper pH
	Resistance or buffer column too high
	Aortic outflow restricted or occluded
	Oxygenator too high relative to the heart
	Temperature too high
	Spontaneous frequency too low
Arrhythmias	Impure water
	Contaminated tubing or glassware
	Errors in perfusate preparation
	Irritation of ventricular tissue by intraventricular probe
	Improper ligation of left atrium to cannula, constriction of coronary artery
	Misalignment of left atrial inflow cannula
	Obstruction in aortic outflow line, impeding coronary flow
	Pacing frequency not sufficiently faster than the spontaneous frequency
	Inappropriate settings on the stimulator
Spontaneous rate regular but too low or high	Impure water
	Contaminated tubing or glassware
	Errors in perfusate preparation
	Temperature too low or high
	Too much atrial tissue ligated or dissected (low frequency)

Observation	Possible causes
Diastolic left ventricular pressure too high	Impure water, insufficient oxygenation
	Contaminated tubing or glassware
	Restricted coronary flow
	Gas pressure too high in closed system
	Temperature too low
Aortic and left ventricular pressures match	Disturbance in the integrity of the aortic semilunar valve by aortic cannula, aortic pressure probe, or intraventricular catheter
Aortic pulse pressure too high or low	Inappropriate volume in compliance chamber

8.   Summary

The strengths of the working rat heart preparation include its proven utility for the study of intact left ventricular function, metabolism, and responsiveness to cardioactive drugs. It allows the quantification of these measurements under rigidly controlled conditions of perfusate composition, external (hydraulic) workload, and contraction frequency, in the absence of confounding variables which may be encountered *in vivo*. Most heart perfusion systems can be categorized as either "open" or "closed," with the major difference being the method of perfusate oxygenation and whether or not the perfusate contains albumin. Either system can be used to study basal mechanical function or responsiveness to cardioactive agents, while the closed system is most often used for studies of cardiac metabolism and is required for perfusion with fatty acids. The stability of the preparation as well as the validity of direct and derived measurements — such as ventricular and aortic pressures, time intervals, rates of pressure rise and fall, and coronary and aortic flows — depend significantly on heart size, the dimensions of aortic and left atrial cannulas, ambient and perfusate temperature, perfusate composition, the extent of perfusate oxygenation, beating frequency, and the design of the volume- and pressure-loading components of the perfusion apparatus. The technique is fairly straightforward, but its successful application requires strict attention to crucial details. Among the most important of these are the following:

1.   The purity of the water used to prepare the perfusate
2.   How thoroughly the components are cleaned
3.   The rapidity of heart isolation and effectiveness of trimming and dissection
4.   The positioning of the cannulas on which the heart is mounted

Recent advancements in digital technology have markedly increased the power of data acquisition and analysis. The basic working heart technique and its variety of applications will very likely continue to be an essential tool for the study of normal and abnormal cardiac physiology, biochemistry, and molecular biology for many years to come.

References

1. Morgan, H.E., Neely, J.R., Wood, R.E., Liebecq, C., Liebermeister, H., and Park, C.R., Factors affecting glucose transport in heart muscle and erythrocytes, *Fed. Proc.*, 24, 1040–1045, 1965.
2. Neely, J.R., Liebermeister, H., Battersby, E.J., and Morgan, H.E., Effect of pressure development on oxygen consumption by isolated rat heart, *Am. J. Physiol.*, 212, 804–814, 1967.
3. Whitmer, J.T., Idell-Wenger, J.A., Rovetto, M.J., and Neely, J.R., Control of fatty acid metabolism in ischemic and hypoxic hearts, *J. Biol. Chem.*, 253, 4305–4309, 1977.
4. Paulson, D.J., Noonan, J.J., Ward, K.M., Stanley, H., Sherratt, A., and Shug, A.L., Effects of POCA on metabolism and function in the ischemic rat heart, *Basic Res. Cardiol.*, 81, 180–187, 1986.
5. Tubau, J.F., Wikman-Coffelt, J., Massie, B.M., Sievers, R., and Parmley, W.W., Improved myocardial efficiency in the working perfused heart of the spontaneously hypertensive rat, *Hypertension*, 10, 396–403, 1987.
6. Flynn, S.B., Gristwood, R.W., and Owen, D.A.A., Characterization of an isolated, working guinea-pig heart including effects of histamine and noradrenaline, *J. Pharmacol. Methods*, 1, 183–195, 1978.
7. Grupp, I.L., Subramaniam, A., Hewett, T.E., Robbins, J., and Grupp, G., Comparison of normal, hypodynamic, and hyperdynamic mouse hearts using isolated work-performing heart preparations, *Am. J. Physiol.*, 265, H1401–H1410, 1993.
8. Taegtmeyer, H., Hems, R., and Krebs, H.A., Utilization of energy-providing substrates in the isolated working rat heart, *Biochem. J.*, 186, 701–711, 1980.
9. Morgan, H.E., Chua, B.H.L., Fuller, E.O., and Siehl, D., Regulation of protein synthesis and degradation during in vitro cardiac work, *Am. J. Physiol.*, 238, E431–E442, 1980.
10. Rodgers, R.L., Depressor effect of diabetes in the spontaneously hypertensive rat: associated changes in heart performance, *Can. J. Physiol. Pharmacol.*, 64, 1177–1184, 1986.
11. Christe M.E. and Rodgers, R.L., Cardiac glucose and fatty acid oxidation in the streptozotocin-induced diabetic spontaneously hypertensive rat, *Hypertension*, 25, 235–241, 1995.
12. Noresson, E., Ricksten, S.-E., Hallback-Nordlander, M., and Thoren, P., Performance of the hypertrophied left ventricle in spontaneously hypertensive rat. Effects of changes in preload and afterload, *Acta Physiol. Scand.*, 107, 1–8. 1979.
13. Biro, G.P., Masika, M., and Korecky, B., Oxygen delivery and performance in the isolated, perfused rat heart: comparison of perfusion with aqueous and perfluorocarbon-containing media, *Adv. Exp. Med. Biol.*, 248, 509–516, 1989.

14. Winslow, R.W., *Hemoglobin-based red cell substitutes*, Johns Hopkins University Press, Baltimore, 1992, 103–106.

15. Bunger, R., Sommer, O., Walter, G., Stiegler, H., and Gerlach, E., Functional and metabolic features of an isolated perfused guinea pig heart performing pressure-volume work, *Pflügers Arch.*, 380, 259–266, 1979.

16. Rodgers, R.L., MacLeod, K.M., and McNeill, J.H., Responses of rat and guinea pig hearts to glucagon: lack of evidence for a dissociation between changes in myocardial cyclic 3',5'-adenosine monophosphate and contractility, *Circ. Res.*, 49, 216–225, 1981.

17. Rodgers, R.L. and McNeill, J.H., Effect of reserpine pretreatment on guinea pig ventricular performance and responsivness to inotropic agents, *J. Pharmacol. Exp. Ther.*, 221, 721–730, 1982.

18. Rodgers, R.L., Chou, H.-N.B., Temma, K., Akera, T., and Shimizu, Y., Positive inotropic and toxic effects of brevetoxin-B on rat and guinea pig heart, *Toxicol. Appl. Pharmacol.*, 76, 296–305, 1984.

19. Bersohn, M. and Scheuer, J., Effects of physical training on end-diastolic volume and myocardial performance of isolated rat hearts, *Circ. Res.*, 40, 510–516, 1977.

20. Segel, L.D., Woliner, M., Miller, R.R., Amsterdam, E.A., Chacko, K.J., Drake, C., Stoll, P.J., and Mason, D.T., Contractility and energetics effects of ethanol and isoproterenol using an improved biologically stable isolated ejecting rat heart system, *Res. Commun. Chem. Pathol. Pharmacol.*, 17, 555–573, 1977.

21. Christe, M.E., Perretta, A.A., Li, P., Capasso, J.M., Anversa, P., and Rodgers, R.L., Cilazapril treatment depresses ventricular function in spontaneously hypertensive rats, *Am. J. Physiol.*, 267, H2050–H2057, 1994.

22. Davidoff, A.J., Pinault, F.M., and Rodgers, R.L., Ventricular relaxation of diabetic spontaneously hypertensive rat, *Hypertension*, 15, 643–651, 1990.

23. Davidoff, A.J. and Rodgers, R.L., Insulin, thyroid hormone, and heart function of diabetic spontaneously hypertensive rat, *Hypertension*, 15, 633–642, 1990.

Chapter 3

Isolated Papillary Muscle Preparation

Joseph M. Capasso

Contents

1. Introduction

An immense amount of useful information has been obtained from the scientific investigation of the pump performance of the heart *in situ*.[1-5] Despite the wealth of literature dealing with global and myocardial functional state, the accurate assessment of the intrinsic contractile performance of the myocardium under these conditions remains difficult and nonprecise. Although much work has been performed to correct for differences in hemodynamic and anatomic variables which are ever present in the intact heart, alterations in neural and humoral regulatory factors, as well as changes in chamber geometry and loading conditions, obfuscate the accurate assessment of the contractile state of the myocardium *in vivo* or *ex vivo*.[4] This situation necessitates that other methodologies be utilized in the evaluation of the intrinsic contractile state of the myocardium. In this regard, procedures and experimental protocols which have been used extensively in the evaluation of the mechanical performance of skeletal muscles have been employed in the characterization of the contractile state of the myocardium.[1-5] As a result of these studies, there has been a considerable increase in the understanding of the physical and chemical factors which directly affect contraction of cardiac muscle. Analysis of the mechanics of myocardial contraction has provided a useful framework for understanding and evaluating the function of not only isolated cardiac muscle but also in the extrapolation of this information to the intact ventricle. By far, the predominant type of experimental preparation utilized for the assessment of intrinsic myocardial contractility is the isolated papillary muscle.[6-16] This preparation was introduced by Abbott and Mommaerts in 1959,[6] but developed as an experimental index of myocardial contractility by Sonnenblick in the early 1960s.[16-29] It was the seminal studies by Sonnenblick that gave rise to an understanding of myocardial performance and global cardiac function in terms of a mathematical description, quantitation, and analysis of its intrinsic contractile state. This early work changed the manner in which basic scientists and clinicians view cardiac function in health and disease. In this preparation, a papillary muscle is removed from the left or right ventricle of an experimental animal and mounted in a muscle bath filled with a buffered physiologic salt solution which mimics the electrolyte concentrations of the blood of that particular species.[6-19]

Strips of endomyocardium have been used to study the mechanics of contraction of cardiac muscle, but these preparations have two major drawbacks: (1) considerable damage results to the preparation in the dissection of these myocardial strips, and (2) the individual fibers are oriented in a nonuniform manner, and the resulting antagonism of the component force vectors serves to temper the interpretation of the accumulated mechanical data. On the other hand, the papillary muscle is particularly suited for the measurement of myocardial contractility since:

1. The papillary muscle is an extension of the endomyocardium.

2. It serves to prevent valvular eversion during contraction and ejection of blood by the heart.

3. All its fibers are oriented in a direction that is parallel to both the long axis of the muscle as well as with force and shortening which occur in this particular cardiac tissue upon contraction.

4. The volume composition of the papillary muscle, i.e., the absolute and relative proportion of nonmyocyte and myocyte compartments, is not different from that of the ventricular wall, and

5. The mechanical response of the papillary muscle to inotropic and chronotropic agents is representative of the entire heart. In addition, little or no damage to the papillary muscle is encountered as a result of dissection of this structure from the ventricular cavity.[20-30]

1.1. Uses of Isolated Papillary Muscle

The papillary muscle lends itself to several different types of investigations. Due to the fact that its size is small enough to allow diffusion of nutrients to its innermost regions, it will remain viable and stable for considerable periods of time, which in some cases may be as great as 6 to 12 h in duration, all of its fibers are oriented in the same direction and in parallel with the long dimension of the muscle, and it has been shown to be representative of the ventricular wall with respect to function, structure, biochemistry, and metabolism. Over the last 3 decades, the isolated papillary muscle has been employed extensively in the assessment of the myocardial contractile state, transmembrane electrical events, contractile protein enzyme activities, morphometric parameters, and intracellular molecular parameters. The muscle has been used to the greatest extent, however, in the evaluation of the contractile state of the myocardium during normal and pathologic states.[17-19,20-30] It is the use of the muscle in the characterization of the contractile state of the myocardium that is the focus of this chapter.

1.2. Contractility

In order to elucidate the contractile properties of the heart, it is advantageous to place a segment of the cardiac muscle into an oxygenated physiologic salt solution and, with the ends of the muscle fixed, to activate the muscle to contract by an electrical stimulus. The muscle contraction which results is termed an isometric contraction (*iso*, same; *meter*, length), since there is no change in external muscle length during the course of the twitch. The magnitude of the isometric force developed during this type of contraction is dependent upon

the intrinsic contractile state of the tissue and the influence of variables introduced by the experimental protocol (i.e., calcium concentration, frequency of
stimulation, solution temperature, presence or absence of inotropic agents).
The force of contraction which results from this electrically induced twitch
can then be measured by utilizing a force transducer as one of the attachment
points of the muscle. Moreover, the timing of the resultant isometric twitch
(the time to peak isometric force, the time to some point in the decay of
isometric force during force relaxation), and its rate of force development (the
first derivative of force or the rate of force development, +dF/dt, and the rate
of force decay, −dF/dt) can be obtained simultaneously.

Alternatively, muscle shortening can be measured in conjunction with
force development by using a lever system attached to either the other end of
the muscle or to the same end if a combination force/length transducer is
employed (Cambridge Technology, Cambridge, MA). When a constant load
is placed on the muscle and the muscle is allowed to shorten and lift this load
in the same manner as the biceps in the arm functions when we pick up an
object with the hand, an isotonic contraction occurs (*iso*, same; *tone*, load).
The load on the muscle can be varied from no load (i.e., unloaded or zero
load) to a load at which no shortening occurs (i.e., the isometric level) prior
to this isotonic twitch, and a series of afterloaded isotonic contractions can be
obtained. Interestingly, as the load is increased on the muscle, the speed at
which the muscle shortens and the actual amount of muscle shortening
decrease. When the muscle is unloaded or is at zero load, the speed or velocity
of muscle shortening is maximum, and this speed is referred to as V_{Max} and is
oftentimes used as an index of the contractile state of the myocardium.

A very useful preparation of heart muscle for these types of *in vitro*
studies is the papillary muscle, which attaches the wall of the ventricle to
either the tricuspid or the mitral valve and is part of the endocardial layer of
the ventricular wall. The muscle has its fibers arranged in a longitudinal,
parallel fashion, and in small animals such as the mouse, hamster, rat, ferret,
cat, and rabbit it is suitably thin so that diffusion of oxygen *in vitro* is adequate
to allow stable function and to avoid hypoxic damage to the core of the
tissue.[16-19] As has been mentioned, during the cardiac cycle the papillary
muscle contracts and shortens and functions to prevent regurgitant flow by
holding the valve closed during the ejection phase of the cardiac cycle.

1.3. Isometric Contractions

Isometric contractions obtained *in vitro* provide information which is directly
applicable to the isovolumic phases of contraction during the cardiac cycle *in
situ*. If, for example, isometric force generation and rate of force generation
are reduced and the timing parameters are increased, more than likely pressure
development in the intact heart will be slow in onset and prolonged in relaxation, and maximum pressure-generating ability of the heart will be reduced.
In the intact animals, these are kinetic and dynamic characteristics which can

result initially in diastolic dysfunction and then later lead to systolic dysfunction and ultimately overt heart failure. Importantly, these abnormalities in the intact heart may be masked initially due to neural or humoral influences, but these external influences are eliminated and/or controlled in the muscle bath, further emphasizing the necessity of the papillary muscle in the assessment of the intrinsic contractile state of the heart.[16-19]

During an experimental protocol in which only isometric contractions are to be examined, a papillary muscle is mounted at both ends to structures which are fixed in space and serve to maintain external muscle length at a constant setting.[20-30] When the papillary muscle is stimulated while held in such a manner, the resultant contraction is termed isometric (same size). Under normal conditions, myocardial tissue (i.e., the papillary muscle) is not fully activated during a single contraction, but the level of activation, which appears to be influenced by the quantity of calcium which is made available to the contractile apparatus, remains constant as long as factors such as contraction frequency, temperature, and the chemical milieu remain unchanged. The amount of force developed by a cardiac muscle which is held at a fixed length is the maximum that the muscle is capable of developing under the conditions set by the experimental protocol (i.e., temperature, bath calcium, stimulation frequency, etc.) and for that muscle length (see Figure 1). This is in direct contrast to skeletal muscle, in which under physiologic conditions the force of contraction is dependent on muscle length to only a small extent and in which the tetanic force of fused twitches is a function of the frequency of nerve impulses. The strength of individual isometric cardiac contractions is readily modified by two major influences. These are a change in initial muscle length, induced by change in the passive stretch of the muscle or preload and a change in contractility or the inotropic state.[16-19]

In all muscle which is striated, however, the actively developed tension or the force developed by the muscle is a function of the initial muscle length. This relationship is much more prominent in cardiac muscle. Myocardial muscle length can be altered by adjusting the initial degree of stretch placed on the resting muscle. When a muscle is stretched in this fashion, a muscle length is found at which the resultant isometric force is maximal when the muscle is stimulated to contract isometrically. This length is termed L_{Max}, the muscle length at which maximum isometric force is obtained. The force or load placed on the muscle which is necessary to stretch the resting muscle to its initial length is termed the preload or resting tension, and the relation between the preload and the length of the resting muscle is called the length – resting tension relation. Preload finds its *in situ* physiologic counterpart in the hemodynamic parameter of end diastolic pressure.[9-15,16-19]

Myocardial isometric tension development can be altered by changing the initial fixed muscle length, and the relation between these length changes and tension variables is expressed by a curve which depicts the changes in force (i.e., stress) vs. the incremental increases in muscle length (i.e., strain). Specifically, the relation between developed isometric tension (i.e., the increment in tension observed during an electrically induced contraction) and initial

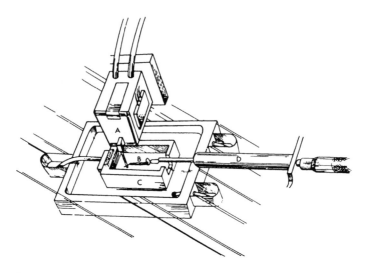

Figure 1

Continuous perfusion myograph. A stainless-steel lever extension of a servo-controlled galvanom-
eter (**A**) is tied to the tendinous end of the papillary muscle (**B**). The nontendinous end of the
papillary muscle is inserted into a spring-loaded stainless steel clip, which forms the rigid
extension of a micrometer (**D**) for the precise adjustment of muscle length. The muscle and its
connections are suspended horizontally in a bath (**C**) for continuous perfusion of solution. (From
Capasso, J.M. et al., *Am. J. Physiol.*, 242, H882-H889, 1992. With permission.)

muscle length set prior to electrical stimulation constitutes the length – active
tension relation. If the initial muscle length is either increased or decreased
from L_{Max}, actively developed isometric force declines. The length – active
tension relation at lengths below L_{Max} is termed the ascending limb of the
curve (*in vivo* it is called the ascending limb of the Starling curve), while at
lengths above L_{Max} it is termed the descending limb of the curve (*in vivo* it is
called the descending limb of the Starling curve).[1-5,16-19]

When a change in contractility is induced, i.e., when the level of activation
is altered by what is termed an inotropic intervention, such as an alteration in
frequency of contraction or by the addition of norepinephrine, the peak force
developed (peak tension) as well as the rate of force development (dF/dt) and
the time to reach peak force (TPF) are changed. Interventions which are
inotropic do not usually alter the relation between muscle length and tension
of the resting or noncontracting muscle, but by definition they do change the
actively developed tension at any given muscle length. It should be noted that
a positive inotropic agent will move the active length tension curve upwards,
resulting in a new active length tension curve which is parallel with the
length–active tension curve in the absence of the inotropic agent. For example,
in the presence of a high calcium concentration in the medium perfusing or
surrounding cardiac muscle, or following the addition of agents such as catecholamines or digitalis glycosides, developed force at any muscle length is
augmented. This upward displacement of the length – active tension curve is
not associated with any change in L_{Max}, i.e., maximum force is still reached

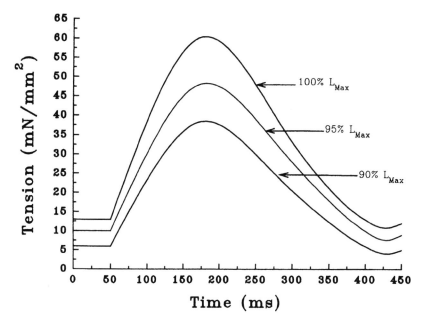

Figure 2

Isometric contractions in which three different muscle lengths have been utilized. To obtain these different muscle lengths and degree of stretch of the muscle, three different preloads or resting tensions have been utilized. As the initial muscle length is increased from 90% L_{Max} to 100% L_{Max}, resting tension rises, as does the peak developed tension. The time to peak tension, however, remains essentially unchanged.

at the same muscle length. In addition, the length – resting tension curve remains unaltered. It should be pointed out that in generating a Starling curve, as muscle length is increased, the time to peak tension (TPF) is either unaltered or is slightly lengthened, while after the augmentation of contractility by the addition of calcium, the time to peak tension is slightly decreased.[16-19]

1.4.   Isotonic Contractions

Isotonic (same load) contractions performed at physiologic loading conditions (i.e., loads which range midway between zero load and the isometric load) are representative of the ejection phases of the cardiac cycle *in situ*. Isotonic contractions provide insight into the ability of the heart to shorten when confronted with a particular physiologic or pathologic loading state and the degree of shortening which will take place at this load. In this way, isotonic contractions are useful indicators of how well the intact heart is able to shorten and eject blood in response to the demands of the body. Equally important is the fact that extrapolation of the speed or velocity of shortening to zero load presents information on the contractile state of the myocardium and indirectly of the contractile state and performance of the intact heart.[1-5,16-19]

In studying the mechanics of cardiac contraction, it is essential to analyze not only isometric contractions but the shortening characteristics of the muscle as well. In order to accomplish this, one end of the papillary muscle is attached to a lever system so that the muscle is free to shorten, and this shortening is measured (Figure 3). A small weight on the opposite end of the lever stretches the passive muscle to a given length; this amount of load is referred to as the "preload" (also called resting force or resting tension), since it is imposed on the inactive muscle prior to the onset of contraction. A stop is then fixed above the tip of the lever near the attachment of the muscle, so that any weight which is added over and above the preload is sensed by the muscle only after the onset of contraction; such added weight is termed the "afterload" (Figure 3) since the weight or load is not imposed on the muscle until after the onset of contraction. In the intact heart, afterload finds its counterpart as systolic arterial blood pressure.

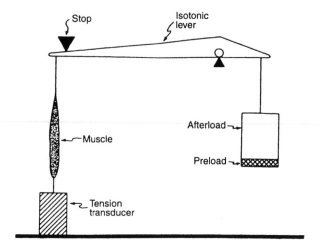

Figure 3

Diagrammatic representation of a system utilized to measure isometric and isotonic papillary muscle contractions. The papillary muscle is placed in a bath of Tyrode solution and stimulated by platinum electrodes placed parallel with its longitudinal axis. The bath and electrodes are not shown for clarity. The lower end of the muscle is attached to an extension from a force transducer, while the upper free end is attached to the end of a lever system which is free to move. The fulcrum of the lever system is shown to the right. Initially the stop is not present. A small weight or preload is placed on the opposite end of the lever and stretches the muscle to a length consistent with its resting length – tension relation. The stop is then fixed above the tip of the lever so that any added weight over and above the preload will not be sensed by the muscle until it attempts to contract. Additional loads or afterloads can be added to the preload. Total load equals the sum of the preload and the afterloads. (From Sonnenblick, E.H., *Fed. Proc.*, 21, 975, 1962. With permission.)

When a papillary muscle is made to contract against an afterload, it first develops force until the level of the afterload is reached and then proceeds to shorten by lifting the preload and afterload (total load) (Figure 4). The

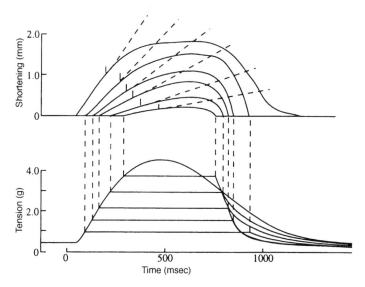

Figure 4

The effects of increasing afterloads on the course of tension development and subsequent muscle shortening. Several superimposed contractions are displayed. As the afterload is increased, the velocity of shortening, represented by the dashed lines in the upper tracings of shortening, and extent of shortening decrease. This depicts the inverse relation between load and velocity or extent of muscle shortening. (From Sonnenblick, E.H., *Fed. Proc.*, 21, 975, 1962. With permission.)

maximum velocity of shortening in each contraction depends on the load, and the relation between the tension (force per unit area) developed and the velocity of contraction is expressed by the load – velocity curve.[16-30] When the load is smallest, the velocity of shortening is greatest. Velocity of shortening with zero load, termed the "unloaded velocity of shortening" or V_{Max}, is not normally measured directly, since the preload is lifted throughout the course of shortening, even with no afterload. Nevertheless extrapolation of the curve back to zero load approximates this maximum velocity of unloaded shortening, termed V_{Max}. When the load is increased to the point at which no external muscle shortening is observed, isometric force is developed at that muscle length.[16-19]

When the initial muscle length is altered by changing the preload, the force – velocity curve is shifted; the velocity of shortening at any given load is changed as is the ability to develop isometric force. Notably, however, V_{Max} is little altered by a change in initial muscle length so that intrinsic contractile state remains relatively unchanged. In contrast, when the contractility, or inotropic state, of the papillary muscle is augmented, the rate of tension development is increased, as is the velocity and extent of shortening with a given load. Developed force is usually augmented as well. The entire force — velocity curve is shifted upward and to the right with an increase in both maximum force and V_{max}.[1-5,16-19]

2. Methodology for Papillary Muscle Preparation

Papillary muscles from the right or left ventricle can be employed for the assessment of myocardial contractility. In large animals (i.e., cat, rabbit, dog) anterior or posterior papillary muscles are removed from the right ventricle, while in smaller mammals (i.e., rat, mouse, hamster, ferret) the left ventricular anterior and/or posterior papillary muscle is usually employed for studies of myocardial contractility.[16-30] Once the heart is removed from the animal, care should be taken in handling the heart, and it is usually best to place the isolated heart in a beaker of heparinized physiologic salt solution. This solution (e.g., Krebs, Tyrode) should be at room temperature and contain heparin in a quantity to prevent clotting for the species under study (e.g., in the rat, heparin is given intraperitoneally at 3000 units/kg body weight). In this way the heart will continue to beat and clear itself of blood, while the heparin allows the coronary arteries to clear and perfuse the tissue with Tyrode's solution.[20-30]

Evaluation of Papillary Muscle Mechanical Characteristics

1. **Select the appropriate animal model.** If, for example, one wishes to study the effects of renal hypertension of the contractile performance of the myocardium, it is not wise to study the right ventricular papillary muscle of a renal hypertensive cat, since the left ventricle is affected to the greatest degree in this condition. It would also not be appropriate to examine the function of the left ventricular papillary muscle from this same animal model, since they would be so large as to limit nutrient transport by simple diffusion. In this case, a better animal model might be the rat or ferret.

2. **Turn on all equipment and have the solution in the muscle bath at the appropriate temperature.** Even solid state devices should be turned on at least 1 h prior to mounting of the muscle. The normal Tyrode solution in the muscle bath should be at the temperature decided upon in the experimental protocol.

3. **Prepare all solutions before the animal is sacrificed.** Time should not be wasted in the sacrifice of the animal, removal of the heart, and excision of the papillary muscle. Papillary muscles are more stable and long-lived *in vitro* if these three procedures are done painlessly, quickly, and without damage to the papillary muscle.

   a. Heparinize the animal

   b. Anesthetize animal (or decapitate, cervical dislocation, etc)

   c. Remove heart and place in normal oxygenated Tyrode's solution containing heparin

   d. Allow heart to beat out (i.e., clear of blood)

   e. Place heart in high potassium (i.e., arresting) Tyrode's solution

4. **Remove the papillary muscle.** The heart and muscle should be kept under the arresting solution throughout the dissection. Care should be taken so as to not stretch the papillary muscle during its removal, because this can be a fatal error in obtaining representative mechanical performance. Overstretch of the muscle at any time results in irreversible damage and depressed function.

   a. Pin the heart to dissecting/petri dish filled with sufficient arresting Tyrode's solution to cover the heart

   b. Cut the heart from base to apex to expose endocardial surface of ventricle of interest

   c. Gently dissect enough tissue from the base of the papillary muscle for mounting

   d. Gently dissect the muscle from the valve by cutting the attached cordae tendinae

   e. Mount the muscle onto the lever/transducer system which is to be put into the muscle bath (clamps, silk, etc.)

   f. Set the resting tension at about 1 g/mm^2 square of cross-sectional area

   g. Stimulate the muscle at 0.1 Hz for at least 1 h equilibration period

   h. Stretch the muscle to determine L_{Max}.

   i. Determine force, timing parameters, and dF/dt at about 10 muscle lengths from slack length (85 to 90% L_{Max}) to L_{Max}

   j. Set muscle at L_{Max} and vary afterload from preload to isometric level while force, shortening, and velocity are obtained

5. **At the end of the experimental protocol:**

   a. Measure the length of the papillary muscle in the bath at L_{Max} (the length of the muscle between the mounting areas at the ends)

   b. Measure the diameter of the papillary muscle in the bath at L_{Max} (the diameter of the muscle should be measured in at least five different regions along the length of the muscle)

   c. Remove the papillary muscle, blot dry, and weigh (the length of the muscle between the mounting areas at the ends)

   d. Cross-sectional area can be calculated from either the length and volume (weight) or from the diameter measurements

      • Papillary muscle cross-sectional area (CSA) can be obtained from muscle length (ML) and muscle weight (i.e., volume or MV; to yield the correct MV, muscle weight must be divided by 1.06, the specific gravity of muscle tissue)

      $$MV = CSA \times ML \text{ or } CSA = MV/ML$$

      yielding CSA in mm^2.

- Muscle cross-sectional area can be derived from the diameter $CSA = \pi(D/2)^2$, where CSA = cross-sectional area in mm^2 and D = diameter in mm.

2.1. Preparation of Solutions

Standard nutrient-fortified physiologic salt solutions containing either glucose and/or fatty acids can be utilized to maintain muscle viability (e.g., Krebs, Tyrode). In some instances, a blood perfusion system is utilized, but this rarely offers any advantage. Solutions should be made up fresh prior to use and concentrated stock solutions of the various salts can be utilized to facilitate this task. Osmolality, calcium, potassium, and pH should be ascertained to ensure that these values are as close to those published for the blood of the species of interest. Initially, these values should be checked daily and then weekly as the investigator becomes more experienced in solution preparation. It is absolutely critical that these parameters be maintained within as small a variability as possibile to ensure the reproducibility of day-to-day studies.[20-30] A recipe for Tyrode's solution follows:

Preparation of Normal and High Potassium Tyrode Solutions

Step 1: Prepare the following salt solutions in the molarities indicated in parentheses. Stock solutions:

> NaCl (4 M)
> MgCl$_2$ (0.5 M)
> NaHCO$_3$ (0.5 M)
> NaH$_2$PO$_4$ (0.5 M)
> KCl (1.0 M)
> CaCl$_2$ (0.5 M)
> dextrose powder.

Step 2: Prepare 2 liters of concentrated (8×) Tyrode solution stock with the following composition:

NaCl (4 M)	550 ml
MgCl$_2$ (0.5 M)	16 ml
NaHCO$_3$ (0.5 M)	384 ml
NaH$_2$PO$_4$ (0.5 M)	57.6 ml

Combine these volumes in a 2-l volumetric flask and bring up to 2000 ml with triple-distilled, deionized water.

Step 3: To make up 1 liter of regular Tyrode solution (calcium concentration = 2.4 mM):

> 125 ml of 8× Tyrode solution stock (step 2)
> 4 ml of 1.0 M KCl
> 1 g of dextrose

Bring up the volume to 995.2 ml
Aerate with 95% O_2 and 5% CO_2
4.8 ml 0.5 M $CaCl_2$

Step 4: To make up 1 liter of high potassium Tyrode solution:
125 ml of 8× Tyrode solution stock (step 2)
30 ml of 1.0 M KCl
1 g of dextrose
Bring up the volume to 995.2 ml
Aerate with 95% O_2 and 5% CO_2
4.8 ml 0.5 M $CaCl_2$

2.2.   Animal Sacrifice and Heart Removal

Prior to anesthetization or just shortly thereafter, animals should be heparinized with sufficient compound (for the adult rat this involves the administration of approximately 3000 U/kg) to prevent clotting throughout the body and particularly in the coronary circulation. Animals should be anesthetized with a compound that does not affect cardiac tissue or which is eliminated rapidly upon removal of the heart, such as chloral hydrate (i.p., 500 mg/kg) (cervical dislocation, decapitation, and ether have also been used to accomplish this objective). Hearts should be rapidly excised by cutting the great vessels at the base of the heart, and the excised heart should be placed in oxygenated physiologic salt solution containing heparin and a normal level of potassium. Under these conditions the heart will contain to beat and clear itself of blood. When the heart appears clear of blood (within 1 to 2 min) it should be placed in another container of physiologic salt solution containing elevated potassium to induce diastolic arrest (in mM: Na^+ 151.3, Ca^{2+} 2.4, K^+ 30.0, Mg^{2+} 0.5, Cl^- 147.3, H_2PO_4 12.0, and dextrose 5.5). This latter solution is often referred to as arresting solution or high potassium Tyrode's.[20-30]

2.3.   Papillary Muscle Removal

Prevent the heart and papillary muscle from drying. In this regard, it is best to keep the heart and papillary muscles under the arresting solution during the dissection. This can be accomplished in a petri dish half filled with beeswax or dental wax to which the heart can be pinned in place. This petri dish and wax combination will allow the investigator to have a miniature dissecting tray. After dissection of the papillary muscle(s), the left and right ventricle and the septum may be prepared for additional assays. In some studies, the right ventricular free wall and the left ventricle (+ septum) are simply weighed after dissection of the papillary muscles.[20-30]

In an ideal study which compares the effect an intervention may have on myocardial contractility, papillary muscles from a control animal and an

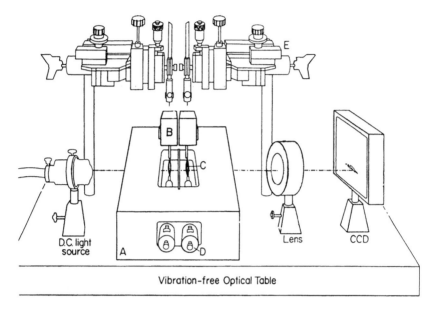

Figure 5
Continuous perfusion myograph in which two papillary muscles (C) can be suspended horizontally for the measurement of isometric and isotonic contractions by the use of two force–length transducers (**B**). Transmembrane electrical events can also be recorded from the muscles simultaneously with mechanical parameters by the use of the two microelectrodes (shown connected to micromanipulators [**E**]). This system has also been configured to record the mechanics of an internal segment of the muscle unencumbered by the potential damage at the ends due to mounting of the muscle in the tissue bath. This is accomplished by a D.C. light source, markers on the muscle, a simple lens, and a Reticon charged coupled device. The entire apparatus rests on a vibration-free optical table which eliminates physical interference in both the horizontal and vertical directions. In this way the mechanical and electrical performance of a papillary muscle can be determined from a control and experimental animal simultaneously and under identical conditions.

experimental animal are removed and suspended side-by-side in a muscle bath (Figure 5). To remove the papillary muscle, the heart is cut from base to apex in such a way as to expose the endocardial surface of the ventricle of interest. The nontendinous end of the papillary muscle is dissected from the ventricle, keeping in mind that enough endomyocardium should remain attached to the papillary muscle that will facilitate attachment of a micrometer assembly for the adjustment of external muscle length. This base of the papillary muscle can then be attached to the end of the micrometer assembly by a spring clip or an appropriate length of surgical silk. The tendinous end of the papillary muscle is attached to a lever system in a similar manner, and this lever is in turn connected to force and/or length transducers to measure isometric and/or isotonic contractions (see below). Commercially available muscle baths can be set up as static baths in which the solution in the bath is not changed during the experiment, or as continuous perfusion baths in which there is a continual wash out of perfusate. In long experiments, static bath conditions may result in a build up of metabolic waste products and inhibit mechanical performance, and thus artifactually affect evaluation of the contractile state of the muscle. In this regard, it is best to continuously perfuse the muscle with the physiologic solution of choice so that wash-out of metabolites can take place. For muscle stability and long life this solution is usually maintained at around 30°C and gassed with 95% O_2 to 5% CO_2. Preparations are stimulated to contract at various rates which are all considerably lower than that observed physiologically. For instance, in rats, this is performed by field stimulation at 0.1 Hz by rectangular depolarizing pulses 10 ms in duration and twice the diastolic threshold in intensity.[8,20-30]

2.4. Determination of Isometric Performance Characteristics

In order to avoid problems due to dimensional variations between papillary muscles from control and experimental animals (and/or between muscles from animals of different sizes, sex, strains and species), force developed by the papillary muscle is described in terms of the cross-sectional area involved in its production.[8,20-30] The expression of force per unit area is tension (τ), which is measured by the units mN/mm^2 (1 g = 9.87 mN). As a papillary muscle is elongated by increasing the preload or resting tension on it, the cross-sectional area (A_o) decreases so that force is generated by a smaller area than at the original length (L_o), and the resultant tension is consequently higher. Thus, tension-generating ability is defined as the force developing capacity (F) per actual instantaneous cross-sectional area (A_i);

$$\tau = F \ (mN)/A_i \ (mm^2)$$

When a uniaxial load is applied to cardiac muscle parallel with its fibers, the tissue responds by deforming and changing its overall length. This strain (ε) is expressed as length change per original length. Thus, changes in length of a muscle from an initial length (L_o), which is assumed to be associated with zero stress, to a new or instantaneous length (L_i) can be described by the relationship which defines the change in linear strain;

$$\varepsilon = \int_{L_o}^{L_i} dL_i/L_i = \ln L_i/L_o \ (mm/mm)$$

This relationship is referred to as the logarithmic or natural strain since the integral $L_i - L_o$ with respect to dL_i is equal to $\ln L_i$. After an equilibration period of 120 min, during which the muscle contracts isometrically at a resting tension of approximately 9.8 mN/mm^2, the passive and active isometric stress-strain relations are determined by shortening muscle length in approximate 1% steps between L_{Max}, the muscle length where force development is maximal, and 90% L_{Max}. Parameters dependent on muscle length are computed at intervals of 1% L_{Max}.[16-30]

2.5. Determination of Isotonic Performance Characteristics

In isotonic experimentations, a load–velocity relation is obtained by setting muscle length at L_{Max} with an appropriate preload and increasing afterload, in steps from preload to the isometric level while recording force, shortening and velocity. It should be recalled that there is an inverse relationship between load and velocity of muscle shortening and peak shortening that occurs during the isotonic contraction. Peak velocity of muscle shortening is measured at each afterload, and load–velocity curves can be constructed. The maximum velocity of unloaded muscle shortening (V_{Max}) can be determined from the intercept of this curve on the Y axis (i.e., by extrapolation of the load velocity curve to zero load). Isotonic parameters are usually measured at each afterload and compared at identical relative loads [(preload + isotonic afterload)/(preload + isometric developed tension) × 100]. Parameters dependent on muscle load are computed at intervals of 5% relative load.[8,16-19]

2.6. Muscle Normalization

At completion of each experiment, muscle length and muscle diameter at L_{Max} are measured with a reticle in the eyepiece of a dissecting microscope set at a total magnification of ×30. Cross-sectional area (XS) can be calculated from papillary muscle diameter (MD), $XS = 3.14159 \times (MD/2)^2$, assuming that the shape of the papillary muscle is equivalent to a right circular cylinder. Force and the rate of force change are then expressed per unit area of tissue to obtain tension and rate of tension change (i.e., dT/dt). Velocity of muscle shortening is expressed in muscle lengths per second by taking the absolute speed of shortening and dividing this value by the length of the papillary muscle involved in the generation of this shortening.[16-30]

2.7. Potential Problems

2.7.1. Anoxic core

This can be a problem in the evaluation of the mechanical performance of papillary muscles which have a cross-sectional area which is greater than 1.0 to 1.5 mm². Since this area represents a limitation in experiments relying upon simple diffusion for the transport of oxygen and nutrients it is often seen as a potential problem in studies of isolated papillary muscles, particularly those which have a cross-sectional area approaching 2.0 mm^2. The phenomenon of the anoxic core may become more apparent when using large muscles and when the stimulation rate and temperature selected are higher than 30°C and 0.1 Hz. This situation can be recognized if in a muscle with a large cross-sectional area the papillary muscle function (i.e., its ability to generate a certain level of developed isometric force at L_{Max}) declines with time. This can be minimized or avoided in these large muscles if bath temperature and/or stimulation frequency are reduced for the duration of the experimental protocol.[8,16-30]

2.7.2. Nonphysiologic temperature and rate of stimulation

It must always be kept in mind that the interpretation of the mechanical performance of the papillary muscle or its contractile state is reflective of the temperature, calcium, stimulation rate, and other influences that may be present in the muscle bath. Although it is truly an excellent barometer of the intrinsic contractile state of the myocardium, it does not reflect cardiac pump performance in all instances. This may be a result of neural–humoral influences that help to regulate cardiac function *in situ* or amelioration of abnormalities observed in the papillary muscle when the intact heart is studied due to the higher heart rate, body temperature, and serum electrolyte concentrations that exist in the intact animal. These caveats should be kept in mind and warn investigators to be cautious in their extrapolation of mechanical information derived from the papillary muscle to global cardiac function in the intact animal.[20-30]

2.7.3. Damage to the ends of the preparation

In mounting the papillary muscle to the devices utilized in the measurement of force and/or length, there is some degree of damage to the tissue, particularly at the end of the muscle. This damage may add stray compliance into the system and can conceivably affect some of the passive properties of the muscle and may even affect the timing of muscle contraction. Although peak developed force levels should be unaffected by this damage, this problem can be circumvented if the mechanic performance of an internal segment of the papillary muscle is evaluated.[16-19]

References

1. Bern, R.M. and Levy, M.N., *Physiology*, Mosby Year Book Publishers, St. Louis, 1993.
2. Honig, C.R., *Modern Cardiovascular Physiology*, Little, Brown, Boston, 1988.
3. Hurst, J.W., *The Heart*, McGraw-Hill, New York, 1987.
4. Rushmer, R.R., *Cardiovascular Dynamics*, W.B. Saunders, Philadelphia, 1976.

5. Wynn, J. and Braunwald, E., The cardiomyopathies and myocarditis, in *Heart Disease: A Textbook of Cardiovascular Medicine*, Braunwald, Ed., W.B. Saunders, Philadelphia, 1987.

6. Abbott, B.C. and Mommaerts, W.F.H.M., A study of inotropic mechanisms in the papillary muscle preparation, *J. Gen. Physiol.*, 42, 533–551, 1959.

7. Asokan, S.K., Frank, M.J., and Witham, A.C., Cardiomyopathy without cardiomegaly in alcoholics, *Am. Heart J.*, 84, 13–18, 1972.

8. Bing, O.H.L., Matsushita, S., Fanburg, B.L., and Levine, H.J., Mechanical properties of rat cardiac muscle during experimental hypertrophy, *Circ. Res.*, 28, 234–245, 1971.

9. Brady, A.J., Time and displacement dependence of cardiac contractility: problems in defining the active state and force-velocity relations, *Fed. Proc.*, 24, 1410–1420, 1965.

10. Brady, A.J., Onset of contractility in cardiac muscle, *J. Physiol. (London)*, 184, 560–580, 1966.

11. Brady, A.J., Active state in cardiac muscle, *Physiol. Rev.*, 48, 570–600, 1968.

12. Brooks, W.W., Bing, O.H.L., Blaustein, A.S., and Allen, P.D., Comparison of contractile state and myosin isozymes of rat right and left ventricular myocardium, *J. Mol. Cell Cardiol.*, 19, 433–440, 1987.

13. Brutsaert, D.L. and Sonnenblick, E.H., Force-velocity-length-time relation of the contractile elements in heart muscle of the cat, *Circ. Res.*, 24, 137–149, 1969.

14. Brutsaert, D.L., Parmley, W.W., and Sonnenblick, E.H., Effects of various inotropic interventions on the dynamic properties of the contractile elements in heart muscle of the cat, *Circ. Res.*, 27, 513–522, 1970.

15. Brutsaert, D.L., Claes, V.A., and Sonnenblick, E.H., Velocity of shortening of unloaded heart muscle and the length tension relation, *Circ. Res.*, 29, 63–75, 1971.

16. Sonnenblick, E.H., Mechanics of myocardial contraction, in Briller, S.A. and Conn, H.L. Eds., *The Myocardial Cell: Structure, Function and Modification*, University of Pennsylvania Press, Philadelphia, 1966, 173–250.

17. Sonnenblick, E.H., Determinants of active state in heart muscle: force, velocity, instantaneous muscle length and time, *Fed. Proc.*, 24, 1396–1409, 1965.

18. Sonnenblick, E.H., Force-velocity relations in mammalian heart muscle, *Am. J. Physiol.*, 202, 931–939, 1962.

19. Sonnenblick, E.H., Active state in heart muscle: its delayed onset and modification by inotropic agents, *J. Gen. Physiol.*, 50, 661–676, 1967.

19a. Sonnenblick, E.H., *Fed. Proc.*, 21, 975, 1962.

20. Capasso, J.M., Palackal, T., Olivetti, G., and Anversa, P., Left ventricular failure induced by long-term hypertension in rats, *Circ. Res.*, 66, 1400–1412, 1990.

21. Capasso, J.M., Sonnenblick, E.H., and Anversa, P., Calcium channel blockade prevents the progression of myocardial contractile and electrical dysfunction in the cardiomyopathic Syrian hamster, *Circ. Res.*, 67, 1381–1393, 1990.

22. Capasso, J.M., Palackal, T., Olivetti, G., and Anversa, P., Ventricular remodeling-induced severe myocardial dysfunction in the aging rat heart, *Am. J. Physiol.*, 259, H1086–H1096, 1990.

23. Capasso, J.M., Li, P., Guideri, G., and Anversa, P., Left ventricular dysfunction induced by chronic alcohol ingestion in rats, *Am. J. Physiol.*, 261, H212–H219, 1991.

24. Capasso, J.M., Malhotra, A., Scheuer, J., and Sonnenblick, E.H., Myocardial biochemical, contractile and electrical performance after imposition of hypertension in young and old rats, *Circ. Res.*, 58, 445–460, 1986.

25. Capasso, J.M., Strobeck, J.E., Malhotra, A., Scheuer, J., and Sonnenblick, E.H., Contractile behavior of rat myocardium after reversal of hypertensive hypertrophy, *Am. J. Physiol.*, 242, H882–H889, 1982.

26. Capasso, J.M., Puntillo, E., Olivetti, G., and Anversa, P., Differences in load-dependence of relaxation between the left and right ventricular myocardium as a function of age in rats, *Circ. Res.*, 65, 1499–1507, 1989.

27. Conrad, C.H., Brooks, W.W., Robinson, K.G., and Bing, O.H.L., Impaired myocardial function in spontaneously hypertensive rats with heart failure, *Am. J. Physiol.*, 260, H136–H145, 1991.

28. Edman, K.A.P. and Nilsson, E., Mechanical parameters of myocardial contraction studies at a constant length of the contractile element, *Physiol. Scand.*, 72, 205–219, 1968.

29. Fein, F.S., Capasso, J.M., Aronson, R.S., Cho, S.C., Nordin, C., Green, B., Sonnenblick, E.H., and Factor, S.M., Combined renovascular hypertension and diabetes in rats: a new preparation of congestive cardiomyopathy, *Circulation*, 70, 318–330, 1984.

30. Rouleau, J.L., Paradis, P., Shenasa, H., and Juneau, C., Faster time to peak tension and velocity of shortening in right versus left ventricular trabeculae and papillary muscles of dogs, *Circ. Res.*, 59, 556–561, 1986.

Chapter 4

Isolated Atrial Preparations

M.K. Pugsley, E.S. Hayes, and M.J.A. Walker

Contents

0-8493-3332-6/97/$0.00+$.50
© 1997 by CRC Press, Inc.

1. Introduction

1.1. Overview

Isolated tissue preparations have been the cornerstone of the physiological and pharmacological evaluation of substances such as hormones and autacoids, as well as natural and synthetic drugs. However the extrapolation of drug effects on isolated tissue preparations to the whole animal can be limited by the complexity of mechanisms present in intact animals. Nonetheless, assessment of the pharmacological action of drugs in isolated tissues is an essential step in explaining the actions of a drug and in guiding further studies in intact animals.[1] Continuing advances with *in vitro* techniques help maintain their value, especially in terms of explaining drug actions from a cellular to an organ level, and eventually to the whole animal.

The cardiovascular system is a rich source of tissues for *in vitro* studies. Some of the most widely used cardiac preparations are various isolated atrial tissues.[2] These preparations may involve the entire atria (both right and left), single atria (right or left), strips of tissue taken from various parts of atria, and even single isolated atrial cells. Intact atrial preparations are particularly useful in assessing cardiac function in terms of beating rate, force of contraction, membrane potentials (ion channel behavior), and biochemical activity (metabolism, second messenger production, etc.). Strips can be obtained from specialized tissue, such as the sinoatrial node, or from adult atrial tissue in general.

The pharmacological actions of drugs in the atria may be studied at a molecular, electrophysiological, biochemical, and physiological levels. This diversity of methods for the study of atria is important since the variety and distribution of ionic currents within and between species are considerable. Therefore, the type of atrial preparation used when attempting to study problems concerning drug actions or cardiac function must be carefully considered.

Whole atria and atrial strips are often used to study the effects of drugs (inotropes, antiarrhythmics) and second messenger mechanisms, since in this tissue it is relatively easy to measure levels of intracellular second messengers such as cyclic-AMP and IP_3[3] and study contractility.

1.2.   Atrial Anatomy

In adult mammalian species the right atrium is thinner, has a large, broad, triangular appearance, and may be larger than the left atrium. The left atrium, in contrast, tends to be narrow, constricted, and tube-like in appearance and has thicker walls than the right atrium. The two atria are separated by an interatrial septum.

The right atrium contains many important anatomical structures necessary for cardiac conduction and coronary circulation (see Figure 1). The sinoatrial node, which lies near the junction of the right atrium and the superior vena cava, is responsible for pacemaker activity in the heart.

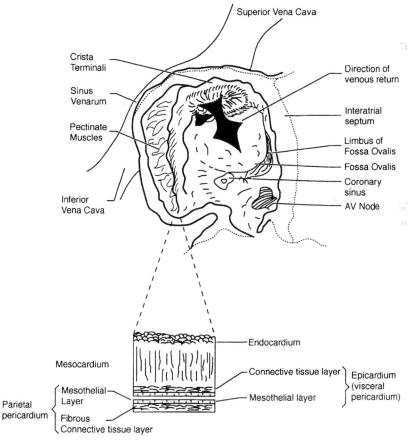

Figure 1

View of the inner aspects of right atrium. In this figure the position of the major anatomical features on the endocardial surface of the right atrium are shown together with a cross-section of the atrial wall.

Ultrastructurally, the atria are not homogeneous. In addition to working atrial cells, the atrium contains P cells (associated with the sinoatrial node), transitional cells (which are the only link between P cells and the remainder of the myocardium), and atrial Purkinje fibers (which comprise the internodal conduction tracts in the atrium).[4]

1.3.   Atrial Physiology and Biochemistry

The role of the atrium is to collect blood from the systemic and pulmonary circulation during the period of ventricular filling, diastole. The intrinsic rhythmicity of the sinoatrial and atrioventricular nodes, plus the conduction of impulses over the atria, allows for the proper coordination of atrial emptying (atrial systole) and ventricular filling (ventricular diastole).

Autonomic neurotransmitters such as norepinephrine (NE) and acetylcholine (ACh) affect atrial automaticity by acting upon receptors, which in turn modulate ionic currents responsible for generation of the cardiac action potential. It should be noted that receptors (and nerves) for the above neurotransmitters are found throughout the atrium. When atrium or atrial tissue is isolated from the heart, the process of isolation leaves the nerve endings of the autonomic nervous system intact. Thus, in isolated atrial tissue there are viable nerve endings containing ACh and NE as well as neuropeptide cotransmitters such as neuropeptide Y and other nonadrenergic-noncholinergic (NANC) neurotransmitters which are functionally significant in the modulation of autonomic tone. In isolated atrial tissue it is possible to release these transmitters and cotransmitters by field stimulation (see later).

1.4.   Atrial Pathology and Clinical Relevance

The functioning of atria is dependent upon many factors such as innervation, age, and circulating hormones, and therefore pathological changes in any of these can result in altered atrial function.

Atrial pathology can result from a variety of biochemical, physical and electrical abnormalities. Such abnormalities are manifest in a wide variety of disorders. Pathological changes related to anatomical (physical) abnormalities of the atrium include, atrial hypertrophy, mitral and tricuspid valvular insufficiency, and atrial septal defects. More often than not these physical pathologies lead to a disturbance of contraction and rhythm.

1.5.   Relevant Atrial Pharmacology

The atria contain numerous membrane bound receptors and ion channels which are targets for a large number of different drugs.[5] Atrial receptors which have been identified both pharmacologically and biochemically include those for peptides (e.g., atrial naturetic factor), autacoids (e.g., histamine, prostaglandins), hormones (e.g., thyroxine, ACTH), neurotransmitters (e.g., NE, ACh), and nucleotides (e.g., adenosine). However, some of these receptors may only play a significant role under limited physical or pathological conditions.

The main area of interest in pharmacological studies which use atrial preparations is in drugs which either alter contractility and/or rate, and rhythm. Neurotransmitters and hormones may alter contractility (inotropism) and often alter rate (chronotropism) and/or rhythm of atria. Thus, agonist and antagonist drugs may increase, or decrease, force and rate. For example, stimulation of atrial beta-adrenoceptors (β_1) results in elevation of the second messenger cyclic-AMP, and subsequent phosphorylation of proteins. This, in turn, results in an increase in calcium current and enhanced calcium binding to the sarcoplasmic reticulum, producing an increase in contractility. On the other hand, inhibition of the Na/K-ATPase by cardiac glycosides (such as digitalis) results in an elevation of intracellular calcium and positive inotropism. Agents which promote (caffeine), or inhibit (ryanodine), the release of calcium from the sarcoplasmic reticulum will augment or attenuate, respectively, atrial contractions.[6]

2. Methods

2.1. General Overview of Methodologies

The following is a brief overview of the methods that can be used to examine the activity of isolated atria. It is intended to help in understanding the equipment required to perform such studies.

2.1.1. Mechanical

The mechanical activity of intact atria, and atrial tissue, can be assessed in various ways and under a variety of loads. Since atrial contraction has evolved to reduce atrial volume, rather than to develop pressure, it is physiologically more relevant to measure contraction under isotonic (same tension or force) rather than isometric (same length or displacement) conditions, although auxotonic (simultaneous force and length changes with time) conditions are probably most physiological.[7] Measures of myocardial contractility include changes in force (or tension), length, contraction and relaxation times. Measurement of the velocity of muscle contraction and relaxation (length/time changes) are useful indices of myocardial contractility.[8]

2.1.2. Biochemical

Biochemical methods for studying atrium are extensive. Depending upon the sensitivity of the methods used, biochemical techniques can be applied from tissue as small as single isolated cells to whole atria. However, the problem with many biochemical techniques is that they are essentially destructive in nature, since they require the chemical processing of tissue in order to obtain the chemical of interest.

In some situations nondestructive methods can be used. Thus oxygen utilization of atrial tissue can be measured by a variety of techniques. In a similar nondestructive manner, the concentration of free calcium in cardiac cells can be assessed by the use of calcium-sensitive dyes, such as Fura-2. Currently, techniques such as nuclear magnetic resonance (NMR) can be used to determine myocardial concentrations of high energy phosphates (ATP, ADP) and pH in isolated whole hearts.[9] Presumably such techniques will become available for use with atria.

2.1.3. Electrophysiological

Electrical activity can be measured in atrial tissue by a variety of techniques. Electrograms and monophasic action potential recordings can easily be obtained from atrial tissue. These are probably poor alternatives to the use of intracellular microelectrodes. Intracellular potentials can be recorded from whole atrium or from a variety of atrial preparations using routine techniques. If the mechanical activity of the preparation makes recording difficult, floating electrodes can be used.

In the past, atrial trabeculae were used for voltage clamp studies, but such use has now been superseded by patch-clamp techniques. Isolated atrial cells can be used for whole-cell patch-clamp and single channel studies.[3]

2.2. Uses and Limitations

2.2.1. Reproducibility (sources of variation)

In most cases, recordings of contractility and rate of isolated atrium of rat, guinea pig, and rabbit are very reliable and the precision of measurements good. In part, this is due to similarities in source of animals, since variability in the size of the animal will affect the size of atria. Such factors are of less importance in strip preparations since, in such cases, standard sized strips can be cut from dissimilar starting materials. The weight of such preparations should be calculated at the end of an experiment.

Poor reproducibility of experimental results with respect to drug action on isolated tissue may be due to instability of the drug or chemicals used. For example, catecholamines are highly susceptible to oxidation, alkaline pH, and photodegradation. It is important that an investigator is always familiar with the lability and solubility of all the drugs and chemicals used. When the drug is not readily soluble an added complication is the use of solubilizing agents. Addition of drugs, dissolved in solutions other than the bathing solution, to an atrial bath can result in precipitation and variable concentrations.

A common problem associated with variability in the use of isolated atrial preparations is the conditions under which cardiac contractility is assessed since the ionic environment of the preparation will affect the contractile state. For example, edema within isolated atrial preparations can cause swelling and changes in length-tension curve and contractility. In such cases it may be beneficial to use osmotic agents such as dextran to limit tissue edema.

Temperature also influences variability. Cooler temperatures are beneficial from a metabolic standpoint and reduce variability, but it is difficult to decide which low temperature to use. For atria from warm-blooded animals temperatures below 25°C appear to fundamentally alter physiology and biochemistry. At higher temperatures (25 to 30°C), drug interactions with receptors and ion channels are probably different from those at 37°C.

2.2.2. Species

It should be noted that there are differences in the type and distribution of ionic currents within and between atrial tissue and that these differences also vary among species. These differences can become important in the assessment of the pharmacological action of drugs, or other interventions. Thus for someone interested in the study of specific bradycardiac agents, i.e., those which block transient outward (Ito) potassium currents, rat atria will be of more use than those from the guinea pig since in the rat this is the dominant repolarizing current in the atria. Tedisamil is such an agent and is more bradycardic in rat atria as compared with guinea pig atria. Figure 2 is an example of the actual records obtained from a rat atrial preparation and shows that tedisamil, an Ito blocker, caused bradycardia and increased contractions.

Differences in the metabolic function of different atrial preparations should be taken into consideration when deciding which preparations and conditions are appropriate. For example, in terms of metabolism and contractility, rat atrial preparations are less susceptible to conditions of hypoxia and raised extracellular potassium, but more to reduced pH, than isolated atrial preparations from guinea pigs and rabbits. Thus for experiments involving the study of ischemia, the choice of species for *in vitro* models will clearly have implications in the assessment of drug action.

2.3. Analysis and Statistics

There are a number of factors which are critical to the analysis (numerical and statistical) of data from studies in general, and atrial studies in particular. These factors include:

1. Identification of sources of variance
2. Identification and normalization for co-variance
3. Adequacy of sampling
4. Transformation of data
5. Dose (concentration) – response studies for drug action

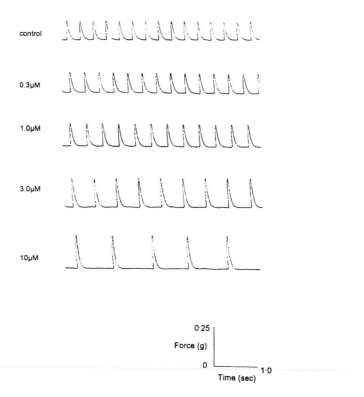

Figure 2
Individual records of contractions of rat isolated right atrium beating spontaneously (control) and in the presence of the transient outward (Ito) potassium channel blocker, tedisamil (0.3–10.0 μM). Note that the positive inotropic effect of tedisamil is not accompanied by a prolongation of contraction.

Factor 1 is considered below. Normalization for sources of covariance means correcting data for identified sources of variability. Thus it is obvious that larger atria will produce greater contractions. The problem is, how to correct data for such factors? Contractile force can be normalized to the weight, surface area, or actin/myosin content of the preparation, for example. The best normalization procedure reduces the quotient of mean/variance to its lowest value, but the best normalizations are often the most tedious (e.g., estimation of actin/myosin control vs. wet weight of atria). However, careful consideration given to normalization repays the investment in terms of improved precision.

The problem of adequacy of sampling is to keep sample size "n" as low as possible while retaining the precision required for most efficiently establishing statistical significance. It is often assumed that the value of "n" should be number of atria used and not the number of tissue samples used. However, the true statistical value of "n" is set by the largest source of variance, be it sample, or atria.

There is great resistance to transforming data (e.g., using the log or square root of data rather than raw data). However, if data do not fit a normal

(Gaussian) distribution they cannot be subjected to parametric statistical tests.[10] On the other hand, simple mathematical transforms (log, square root, sine, cosine, arctan) can convert data to a normal distribution[11] and such normalization procedures are an integral part of many statistical software packages.

The analysis of data from isolated atrial studies should be organized in such a manner so as to aid subsequent statistical analysis. The basic ANOVA procedure comes in many variants, each designed to cope with factors such as covariants (e.g., ANCOVA), or where each variable is measured repeatedly. The techniques available to deal with the latter problem (i.e., repeated measures) have been carefully considered recently.[12] ANOVA, or its variants, are available on many statistical software packages (e.g., NCSS©*, SYSTAT©**, or SPSS™***).

3. Equipment Required

3.1. Physiological Solutions

A number of physiological solutions are available for use with isolated atrial preparations.[13,14] The solutions discussed provide a substitute for blood, which is the physiologically ideal solution with which to perfuse or bathe atrial tissue. However, blood has a number of properties (e.g., clotting and foaming) which make it difficult to use; hence it is rarely used.[15]

Table 1 lists the ionic composition of commonly used mammalian and amphibian physiological solutions for atrial tissue. The table shows that physiological solutions only approximate the ionic concentrations found in plasma. Furthermore, such solutions contain no hormones or proteins, and usually have poor osmotic and oxygen-carrying properties. Complex solutions (which include the addition of insulin and other hormones, metabolic intermediates, etc.) have been described in detail[15] but appear to be no more useful than the solutions described in Table 1.

The oxygen carrying properties of these solutions can be improved by adding oxygen carriers (fluorinated hydrocarbons), while osmotic balance can be improved or maintained by the addition of materials such as sucrose or polyvinylpyrrolidone.[16]

For some solutions, their ionic compositions were established before the concentrations (or more properly activity) of such ions in plasma had been ascertained. In other cases ad hoc changes were introduced in an attempt to obtain more stable preparations. A good example of this is the potassium concentration used in most solutions. In typical bathing solutions it can be as high as 5.9 mM (Krebs-Henseleit), which is much higher than the 3.6 mM found in blood. The use of such high concentrations of potassium is associated

---

*   Registered Trademark of Dr. J.L. Hintze, Kaysville, UT.
**   Registered Trademark of SYSTAT, Inc., Evansville, IL.
*** Registered Trademark of SPSS, Inc., Chicago, IL.

TABLE 1
Ionic Composition of Typical Physiological Solutions Suitable for Atrial Tissue as Compared with Plasma Levels of Ions

Solution	Cations					Anions				Urea	Glucose
	Na^+	K^+	Ca^{2+}	Mg^{2+}	Cl^-	HCO_3^-	$H_2PO_4^-$	SO_4^{2-}			
Mammalian											
[Plasma]$_t$	152	3.7	2.7	1.06	114	26.5	1.7	0.69		7.0	5.8
[Plasma]$_i$	150	3.6	1.6	0.76	112	25.7	1.6	0.69		7.0	5.8
[Interstitial]$_i$	147	3.5	1.5	0.72	115	26.3	1.7	0.73		7.0	5.8
Tyrode[a]	149	2.7	1.8	1.05	145	11.9	0.42	0		0	5.6
Locke[a]	159	5.6	2.1	0	167	1.8	0	0		0	11.2
Krebs-Henseleit[a]	143	5.9	2.5	0	128	24.9	1.18	1.64		0	11.0
PIPES	121	3.4	2.5	1.2	130	0	0	0		0	11.1
Amphibian											
[Plasma]$_t$	104	2.5	2.3	2.9	74	25	3.1	0.10		NR	8
Ringer	111	1.9	1.1	0	114	2.4	0	0		0	2.3
Adrian	115	2.5	1.8	0	121	0	3.0	0		0	0
Horowitz[b]	111	3.4	2.7	0	0	0	0.17	0		0	0

Note: All concentrations are in mM (NR = not reported). Typical total [Plasma]$_t$ and ionized [Plasma]$_i$ ion concentrations in mammalian plasma as well as ionized ion concentration in interstitial fluid [Interstitial]$_i$ are provided for comparison.

[a] The pH for Tyrode, Locke, and Ringer solutions depends upon CO_2 content of the gassing mixture used (usually 95% O_2 and 5% CO_2). PIPES [Piperazine-N,N'-bis-(2-ethanesulfonic acid)] buffer requires 100% oxygenation. Krebs-Henseleit contains 2.0 mM pyruvate.

[b] To buffer solution add NaOH to obtain pH 7.4, then 2.0 mg/l NaH_2PO_4 and a sufficient amount of Na_2HPO_4 to obtain a final buffered solution pH of 7.4.

with fewer arrhythmias in whole hearts and isolated tissue preparations. Similarly, the activity of calcium ions in physiological solutions is often double that found in plasma. In some modified solutions EDTA and EGTA (calcium chelating agents) have been used to chelate cations.[17] A further complication of some solutions is the use of bicarbonate buffers which rely on mixed gas bubbling (95%O_2 + 5%CO_2) to maintain a pH of 7.4. This results in an inherent instability of pH, which depends critically upon CO_2 levels. Thus all of the available solutions are far from ideal. The best approach is to use the most physiologically suitable solution for the experimental tissue being used.[15,18,19]

The basic principles of chemistry dictate that it is best to follow a certain order in the preparation of solutions such as those described in the table. Each salt must be completely dissolved in distilled water to prevent salt crystallization or precipitates. Calcium chloride in solution is *always* added last, subsequent to a final pH (7.4) determination. Glucose is usually added immediately prior to experimental use of a previously prepared solution.

A further problem with physiological solutions is their inability to provide nutrition to the medial cell layers of an atrial preparation. As theorized by Hill, and shown in studies by Krebs,[20] nutrients and oxygen penetrate only the outermost layers of cells by simple diffusion. Anoxia, and the resulting death of middle layer cells with subsequent sequelae, may affect the ability of different layers of cell to propagate action potentials and contract in a manner similar to that which occurs in intact animals.[21]

3.2. Isolated Tissue Baths

The type of tissue bath used for isolated atrial preparations depends upon the type of preparation used and responses measured. A simple vertical tissue bath of 5 to 25 ml volume is usually sufficient for studying beating rate and contraction in whole atria. Both the bath and fluid reservoir should be temperature controlled and oxygenated. Most vertical organ baths are constructed such that gas and reservoir fluid inlets enter from the bottom with a run-off outlet at the top. The bath drainage outlets should be located below gas and reservoir fluid inlets to allow for uncontaminated replacement of bathing fluid. Drainage should be connected to a vacuum for rapid exchange and for adjusting the volume of bathing solutions (see Figure 3).

For experiments involving microelectrodes, a horizontal tissue bath is required. With this type of tissue, bath microelectrodes (held by micromanipulators) may easily be inserted into atrial cells. Microscopes, mounted either underneath or above the bath are used to visualize tissue. The flow and direction of bathing solution can be controlled with a perfusion cannula connected via a manifold (with low dead space) to multiple solution reservoirs such that local flow across a microelectrode-impaled cell can be rapidly (<2 s) and completely changed. Similarly, gasses used to bubble perfusate can be controlled by needle-valves placed at the headstage of the gas source and with an outlet at the level of the tissue bath. The perfusate solution is more effectively aerated, and less tissue disruption occurs with fine water-saturated bubbles than with large ones. Indirect oxygenation, i.e., bubbling the solution at some distance from impalement, is only effective for studies of the electrophysiology of surface atrial cells. Direct bath oxygenation is preferred, especially for functional studies, since a higher oxygen content in the bathing solution ensures better tissue oxygenation

When small force electrical recordings are made from atrial tissue it is important to limit mechanical movement, since this introduces electrical artifacts, may dislodge electrodes, and may decrease resolution. Many specialized damping elements (multilayered, fiber-impregnated pads), epoxy resin stabilizing slabs, tables, and antivibration stands can be purchased to provide a vibration-free environment.

3.3. Transducers

Transducers, by definition, are devices used to convert one form of energy to another, more usable, form. The usual atrial response being measured is the development of force, or work (see Table 2 for units of work). A large number of force transducers with wide ranges of sensitivity are commercially available, which use piezoelectric, optical, or resistive devices to convert atrial force into voltages or current.[2,7] Table 3 describes several different makes and models of isometric and isotonic force transducers and compares some of their properties.

TABLE 2
Physical Units for Force-Displacement Transducers
Used with Isolated Atrial Preparations

Measure	Physical equation(s)	Unit(s)
Force (F)	$m \times a$	$kg \times m/s^2$ = Newton (N)
Work (W)	$F \times d = m \times a \times d$	$N \times m = kg \times m^2/s^2$ = Joule (J)
Power	$W/t = (F \times d)/t$ $= (m \times a \times d)/t$	J/s = Watt
Frequency (F)	oscillations/t	Hertz (Hz)

Note: The above table uses SI abbreviations where m = mass (kilogram),
a = acceleration, t = time (second), and d = distance (meter).

3.4. Stimulating and Recording Electrodes

Bipolar electrodes are adequate for stimulation of isolated atrial preparations and for recording atrial electrograms. More sophisticated electrodes are required for recording extracellular and intracellular potentials. Stainless steel electrodes may be adequate for stimulation of isolated atria but are not really suitable for recording purposes.[22] When stimulating isolated atrial preparations, a reduction in the distance between the electrodes reduces the size and variability of the threshold current required to stimulate muscle and thereby limits the risk of tissue damage. The accurate placement of stimulating electrodes, within 1 to 2 mm, can be achieved through the use of small (27G) needles for inserting electrodes into tissue. The use of Teflon*-coated silver wire ensures that focal depolarization occurs only at tip of the electrode and that the remainder of the electrode remains insulated. Heat applied to the Teflon coating can be used to expose a minimum length of bare silver wire. Thus, direct stimulation of atrial tissue preparations is best achieved by focal depolarization of a small area of tissue and is more "physiological" in nature.

Field stimulation of atrial preparations is achieved by applying, with large electrodes, a large current across the entire tissue preparation so as to generate

* Registered Trademark of E.I. duPont de Nemours and Company, Inc., Wilmington, DE.

TABLE 3
Force-Displacement Transducers Used for Atrial Muscle Contraction Measurement

				Isometric		
Manufacturer	Model	Voltage output	Power	Output impedance (Ω)	Linearity	Sensitivity deflection/ gram load
Harvard Instruments	Res. Grade	2 V, D.C.	115 V, 60 Hz	10,000	±1%	0.1–10 μm
Kent Scientific Instruments	TRN001	—	12 V, A.C.	—	1% (0–20 g)	2.54 μm
[a]Grass Instruments	FT03	8 V	—	—	—	0.0005–0.02 mm
World Precision Instr.	Fort100	10 V	—	350	<0.1%	1800 μV/V

				Isotonic		
Manufacturer	Model	Voltage output	Power	Output impedance (Ω)	Linearity	Breakaway torque (g × cm)
Harvard Instruments	Res. grade	±2 V, D.C.	115 V, 60 Hz	—	±1%	0.05
[b]Kent Scientific Instruments	TRN007	—	—	—	—	—
World Precision Instr.	DSPL	16 μV/mm	—	10,000	2%	—
Stoelting	7006	300 μV/mm	5 V, 13 mA	1,500	±2% to ±15° rotation	>0.1

Note: (—) indicates information is not available. Please consult manufacturer for specifics.

[a] Indicates that Grass Instruments supplies three sets of insertable springs which provide four transducer ranges.

[b] This model and its specifics are available with a custom order from Kent Scientific Corp., Litchfield, CT.

a voltage field. The advantages of field stimulation include: (1) less variable electrode-tissue resistance, (2) consistent contractile behavior due to less variability in muscle fiber conduction, and (3) enhanced synchrony of contraction. Due to the low resistance of the bathing solution and relatively small mass of the tissue preparation, large currents are required for field stimulation which result in the generation of heat and possible tissue damage.

Electrical activity in atrial tissue is often recorded as electrograms, or intracellular potentials. There are several assumptions made with respect to recording bioelectrical events using bipolar techniques, while special properties of myocardial muscle activation have important implications. When using bipolar electrodes it is assumed that the electrode contact surface is small and that the distance between the tissue mass, with respect to the tissue excited, is large.[23] Unlike other types of muscle, cardiac muscle does not repolarize until the muscle has been completely activated. Thus, over the distances used to record atrial electrograms, the electrodes will see both activated and inactivated tissue simultaneously. Even though the activity of the tissue closest to the electrode dominates the signal, surrounding tissue also contributes, thus making the three-dimensional structure of the tissue of some importance to electrogram morphology.[24]

3.5. Recording Devices

Equipment designed to record the various electrical and contractile events in isolated atrial preparations usually consists of (1) a transducer or electrode(s), (2) a signal conditioner, (3) a preamplifier (i.e., carrier, AC/DC), and (4) an analog and/or digital recorder (i.e., strip chart recorder, computer), as shown in Figure 3. The following discussion is limited to preamplifiers and recording equipment.

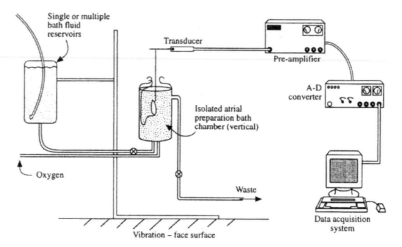

Figure 3

Schematic of apparatus required to record atrial activity. Most transducers require a signal conditioner in order to provide a signal suitable as an input signal for the preamplifier. The analog signal from the preamplifier can be directed to a chart recorder if a hard copy of the analog signal is required.

Preamplifiers allow one to modify the input signal prior to amplification. They usually have high impedance and high gain, characteristics which allow for accurate multiplication, by several orders of magnitude, of the small currents from bioelectrical and biomechanical events in atrial tissue.[25] In most cases preamplifiers are equipped with filters which can be of a high-pass, low-pass, or notch type.[26] The use of combinations of high- and low-pass filters removes troublesome noise and can provide clean and reproducible signals without attenuation of the original signal.

Direct curvilinear ink and paper chart recorders (such as the Grass®* Model 7 Series Polygraph) are the most widely used of recording devices. The variable paper speeds, range, gain, and accuracy of curvilinear chart recorders make it possible to record and analyze most variables associated with the frequency and strength of isolated atrial contraction. Differentiators are especially useful for calculating the first derivative of contraction, with respect to time, for isolated atrial preparations. However, for the greater accuracy needed in quantifying high frequency events such as the action potential, or ionic current transients, digital recording systems are necessary.

Digital recorders may take the form of audio/video tape recorders (PCM based on VCR technology), DAT (digital audio tape), or computer drives. A PCM-based processor combined with video tape recording offers an economical form of on-line data recording.[27] While the various methods of recording each have their specific strengths and weaknesses, there is a need for analog to digital (A/D) conversion. A large number of commercial data acquisition boards are available which take (as an input) analog signals, as voltages, and change these into digital codes for transfer to MS-DOS** or Macintosh*** operating system computers.

Frequency modulation (FM) tape recorders have a voice-over capability which is useful for note-taking during the course of experiments. Such recorders are compatible for use with various types of A/D boards and preamplifiers while the small size and light weight provide convenience.

A wide variety of signal processing hardware and software exists. There are systems which are Macintosh supported, and those which rely on MS-DOS. The choice of software depends upon the available computer and user familiarity with different systems. Software packages such as BIOWINDOW† from Modular Instruments or LabWindows†† from National Instruments are the most flexible of all data handling packages.

4. Methods

The general utility and limitations to the various atrial preparations and techniques available have been outlined previously. The following examines, in detail, the techniques used to record atrial contractions.

---

* Registered Trademark of Grass Instruments Company, Quincy, MA.
** Registered Trademark of Microsoft Corporation, Redmond, WA.
*** Registered Trademark of Apple Company, Inc., Cupertino, CA.
† Registered Trademark of Modular Instruments Corporation, Malvern, PA.
†† Registered Trademark of National Instruments Corporation, Austin, TX.

4.1. Techniques

4.1.1. Small animal whole atrial preparations

For the mouse, rat, guinea pig, and rabbit the following method can be used for the isolation of atrial tissue. Some studies suggest that rabbits between 2 to 3 kg provide uniformly sized atria and less variable contractile differences.[2,5] Large differences in heart size can be avoided by consistent use of similarly sized animals. The animal is given pentobarbitone (65 mg/kg, i.p.) plus heparin (200 U), either administered concurrently or after the anesthetic, by the same route. Once anesthetized, the animal is exsanguinated.

The removal of the heart begins by making a transverse incision at the level of the xyphoid. The general process is described in great detail in the manual by Doring and Dehnert,[15] while Figure 4 gives a diagrammatic representation of the process. Another transverse incision should parallel the diaphragm across the abdominal cavity and not the thorax. This incision exposes the xyphoid process which can be grasped by a pair of tissue forceps and used as an anatomical landmark for the remainder of the surgical procedure. A flap is made of the anterior thoracic wall by cutting through the ribs and chest wall in a cephaled direction to the clavicles, from two extreme lateral points of the initial transverse cut. The anterior chest wall can then be averted so as to expose the heart. This process should take less than 20 s.

The heart is removed from the body cavity by initially opening the pericardial sac and severing the blood vessels (such as the vena cavae) lying superior to the aortic root just beneath the brachiocephalic artery. This is easily performed by using a pair of curved forceps to hold the aorta and cutting above the forceps with surgical iris scissors. Lifting the heart away by the aortic root exposes the remainder of the connective tissue and blood vessels (such as the pulmonary arteries and veins), which can easily be cut without damaging the atrium or sinoatrial node. The heart should be immediately transferred to ice-cold, oxygenated bathing solution, where it beats slowly. The entire process described above takes no longer than 60 to 90 s.

If the heart is then flushed (after the insertion of a cannula into the aorta) with 50-ml ice-cold solution, this washes away the blood in ventricles and atria. This perfusion method is preferred to that of squeezing the heart, since damage is avoided. The atrium are separated from the heart by lifting the atrial appendage and cutting along the atrioventricular sulcus. The atria are placed in oxygenated perfusate solution in a petri dish, and any remaining ventricular or other tissue is trimmed off. Care must be taken not to damage the remaining sinoatrial nodal tissue if the right ventricle is to be used as a spontaneously beating preparation. If the left atrium is used careful dissection of the interatrial septum ensures a nonbeating preparation. The left atrium tends to be more "rugged" than the right and has the added advantage of being easy to pace electrically at suitable frequencies (0.05 to 100 Hz) without interference from spontaneous electrical activity arising from nodal cells.

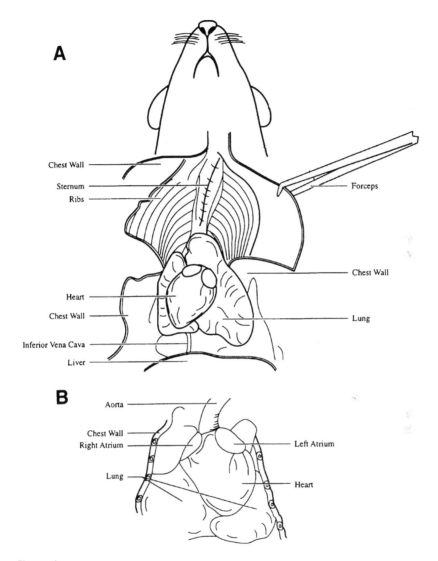

Figure 4
General diagram indicating the approach used to remove the heart from a small animal. The diagram shows how the chest is opened (**A**) and the appearance of the heart once the chest is open (**B**).

The remaining atrial tissue should appear bow-like in appearance when stretched lightly at the ends. Levi (1971) outlines an additional procedure whereby the left atrium can be cut longitudinally producing two "fan-shaped" tissue pieces, the larger of which (usually less than 1 cm^2 depending on the animal species) is used. A suture (usually 3-0 black-braided silk) is made at either or both ends of the atrial tissue as desired. One end can be attached to a hook which is then submersed in an organ bath of appropriate size (usually

25 ml), containing oxygenated solution maintained at 30-35°C. The remaining tie is attached to a force-displacement transducer. The tissue is allowed to equilibrate under isometric tension (usually between 0.25 to 1.5 g) for 30-60 min. The tissue should either remain quiescent (with left atrial preparations) or paced at a frequency established by the experimenter (with right atrial preparations). However, arrhythmias may occur which should subside during tissue equilibration. If they do not, this indicates that the tissue may have been damaged during removal from the body. If the latter is suspected, replace the tissue entirely with a new preparation as it is not recommended that drugs be used to inhibit arrhythmias since this may contaminate the tissue responses to any drugs being examined.

The time provided for initial equilibration of atrial tissue under control conditions is variable, but it is generally considered that 60 min is more than adequate. The resting tension of the preparation can be adjusted repeatedly by simply changing the applied force from the transducer, either during equili-bration or just prior to beginning drug administration. Experience in our laboratory suggests that it is best that the tissue is washed 2 to 3 times with 25 ml of bath solution and tension adjusted at fixed (20 min) intervals during equilibration. Bath solutions should be simultaneously drained and filled by opening the lower fluid inlet valve and upper run-off outlet, respectively, to the bath chamber. Tension is usually increased during equilibration; however, it can be lowered, i.e., one can start from a high resting tension and reduce it until the desired equilibrium tension is obtained. There is little difference in results obtained. Drug administration occurs by directly adding the drug to the bath solution using a syringe or, as discussed above, via a perfusion cannula. Either method allows for an immediate exposure of the tissue to the drug concentration. Drug addition directly to the bath chamber is preferred, in the absence of a perfusion cannula, to actually draining the bath and substituting the bathing solution with a new drug or drug concentration, as the latter may disrupt the equilibrated tension developed by the tissue. Atrial preparations can remain functional for several hours after isolation provided adequate bath oxygenation is maintained. A simple method by which to exam-ine viability is to begin by providing a dose of a neurotransmitter (e.g., 1 μM acetylcholine), wash, equilibrate the tissue, and repeat this at the end of the experiment. If the tissue is viable the response at the end of the experiment should be similar to that at the beginning.

Upon completion of the experiments, the isolated atrial bath chamber should be thoroughly rinsed with 1 to 2 l of distilled water to ensure complete removal of the physiological saline solutions. Electrodes should be cleaned with distilled water and allowed to air-dry. Usually no special cleaning solu-tions are required with this apparatus.

The best technique by definition is that which provides the most repro-ducible responses over the longest duration of observation. Many factors contribute to reproducibility, such as animal species, type of atrial preparation, and standard laboratory practices. In both left and right atrial preparations consistency of either the force of contraction or beating rate (between 75 to

150 beats/min) in right atrium can be used as a marker of equilibrium. Since left atrial beating rate is usually set by external electrical stimulation at a fixed frequency, force of contraction is the only useful indicator for equilibrium in this tissue.

4.1.2. Large animal whole atrial preparations

As mentioned above, whole atrial *in vitro* preparations from cats, dogs and sheep tend to be too thick for adequate oxygenation. Therefore, atrial preparations from these species usually consist of strips of tissue (see below). In any case, removal of atria from these species is often performed under anesthesia.

Several authors have developed techniques for the blood perfusion of isolated dog right atrium by blood from a donor dog.[28] This is a technically demanding and time-consuming preparation requiring surgical skill and good equipment. The dog supplying the blood for perfusion is anesthetized with 30 to 40 mg/kg pentobarbitone i.v. and ventilated with room air. A carotid artery and jugular vein are cannulated together with femoral artery and vein. The carotid artery is used for recording blood pressure. Blood is taken from the femoral artery and returned to the femoral vein.

The dog supplying the isolated atrial tissue is anesthetized and ventilated in the same manner as above. The chest cavity is then exposed by making a parasternal incision and the heart prepared for retrograde perfusion *in situ* by clamping the superior vena cava and inserting a drain into the inferior vena cava. The aorta is cannulated and perfused with cold bathing solution. After the heart has been removed from the chest cavity, while undergoing perfusion, the right circumflex, posterior septal, and anterior septal arteries are cannulated and the atrium dissected free of the remainder of the heart. The cannulated arteries are then connected to the carotid arterial supply of the donor dog via a peristaltic pump. Drainage from the isolated atrium is collected and pumped back to the donor animal via the femoral vein. Anchoring and attachment of the preparation are accomplished in a horizontal tissue bath in a manner similar to that described above. Heparin (500 U/kg, plus 200 U/kg hourly, i.v.) is used to prevent clotting of blood in the isolated atrial preparation. The tissue is washed, as described above, at similar time intervals. Drugs are administered through a side-arm in the perfusion cannulae supplying the blood from the donor dog to the atrial tissue.

4.1.3 Atrial strips (right or left)

As described above, isolated atrial strips are usually obtained from larger species and include human atrial preparations obtained during open-heart surgery. In most cases, narrow strips of atrium are obtained through excision between the anterior vena cava and the atrio-ventricular groove. Usually tissue is obtained from the middle of the atrial wall with cuts parallel to the pectinate muscles. Isolated tissue from human subjects is usually obtained in the form of an approximately 1 cm^2 atrial appendage removed as a part of the cannulation procedure for cardiopulmonary bypass.[28] Atrial strips can be mounted in vertical or horizontal organ baths and attached to an appropriate recording device as described above. Atrial strips are often used in micro-electrode studies of action potentials where they are mounted in horizontal tissue baths. Atrial strips from larger species are also suitable for measurement of atrial contractility.

4.2. Data Obtained

The type of data obtained from isolated atrial preparations depends on which aspect of cardiac function is studied. In the case of contractions and rate, such responses are continuously recorded throughout the duration of the experiment. Such a data stream can either be averaged (as with a tachograph) for rate, or sampled as, and when, considered appropriate. However, other variables can only be sampled in a more punctate manner. For example, to study contractility in terms of length-tension relationship requires that recording is occasionally stopped and the length-tension curve constructed by altering resting tension over a suitable range. Obviously this can only be done a limited number of times.

In electrophysiological studies, it is possible to record electrograms continuously. However, with intracellular studies this is not possible since each impalement only lasts for a limited amount of time, as short as a few seconds or as long as 20 min.

For both mechanical and electrical studies separate contraction and relaxation cycles can be analyzed extensively. Thus for contractions it is possible to measure not only peak contraction but also rate of development of contraction and relaxation.

In determining the direct actions of drugs on atrial function, extensive use is made of concentration-response curves (see Figure 5). Classic examples in isolated whole atria are cumulative dose response curves for isopropylnoradrenaline (IPNA) or acetylcholine. Such curves can be obtained in the presence and absence of other drugs or pretreatment. The responses measured are usually the rate and force of atrial contraction. For example, parallel rightward shifts of the concentration-rate response curve for IPNA with increasing concentrations of a second drug is a good indication of competitive β-antagonism. Similar shifts in concentration-rate response curves for the negative inotropic and chronotropic actions of acetylcholine suggests muscarinic receptor blockade. Concentration-response studies can also be performed in the presence of agents that affect second messenger systems. Normally these studies are carried out in a four-step protocol of (1) dose response curve to standard agent, (2) wash and recovery of tissue to pre-drug values, (3) incubation of tissue preparation with test agent, and (4) repetition of the dose response curve. Ideally a final recontrol curve should also be obtained but this is not always possible.

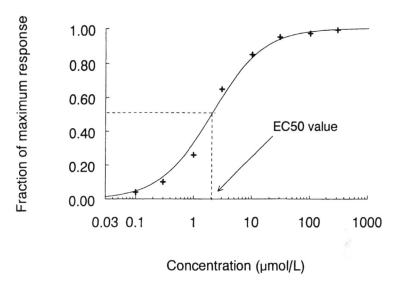

Figure 5

Typical dose response curve. The log concentration is plotted on the abscissa while the fraction of the maximum response is plotted on the ordinate. The effective concentration for a 50% maximum (EC50) response is indicated on the diagram.

5. Summary

This chapter has described a number of available atrial preparations. It provides essential background details on the anatomy, physiology, biochemistry, and pharmacology of atrial muscle and the special mechanical and electrophysiological properties of this tissue. It either outlines, or describes in detail, the procedures and techniques which a researcher may consider using in order to assess atrial function and its response to drugs. Particular emphasis is placed on the problems and sources of variance. We hope that the latter discussion will serve as a guide for improved experimental design which will improve the quality of results.

Acknowledgments

Some of the described studies were conducted with financial support from the Heart and Stroke Foundation of B.C. and Yukon, The British Columbia Health Care Research Foundation, and Rhythm Search Developments, Ltd. M.K. Pugsley is a recipient of a Science Council of B.C. GREAT award and a Personnel Award from the Heart and Stroke Foundation of British Columbia and Yukon.

References

1. Hainsworth, R. and Mary, D., Cardiogenic reflexes, in *Encyclopedia of Human Biology*, vol. 2, Academic Press, New York, 1991, 137.

2. Levy, J.V., Isolated atrial preparations, in *Methods in Pharmacology*, Schwartz, A., Ed., Appleton-Century-Crofts, New York, 1971, chap. 3.

3. Sorota, S. and Boyden, P.A., Electrophysiology of the atrial myocardium, in *Electrophysiology and Pharmacology of the Heart*, Dangman, K.H. and Miura, D.S., Eds., Marcel Dekker, New York, 1991, chap. 6.

4. Berne, R.M. and Levy, M.N., *Cardiovascular Physiology*, C.V. Mosby, St. Louis, 1986, chap. 2.

5. Katzung, B., Evaluation of drugs affecting the contractility and electrical properties of the heart, in *Selected Pharmacological Testing Methods*, Burger, A., Ed., Marcel Dekker, New York, 1968, chap. 6.

6. Northover, B.J., Effects of pretreatment with caffeine or ryanodine on the myocardial response to simulated ischaemia, *Br. J. Pharmacol.*, 103, 1225, 1991.

7. Blattener, R., Classen, H.G., Dehnert, H., and Doring, H.J., *Experiments on Isolated Smooth Muscle Preparations*, Hugo-Sachs Elektronik KG, Freiburg, 1978, chap. 2.

8. Parmley, W.W. and Sonnenblick, E.H., Cardiac muscle function studies, in *Methods in Pharmacology*, Schwartz, A., Ed., Appleton-Century-Crofts, New York, 1971, chap. 4.

9. Garlick, B.P., Radda, G.K., and Seely, P.J., Studies of acidosis in the ischaemic heart by phosphorus nuclear magnetic resonance, *Biophys. J.*, 184, 547, 1979.

10. Wallenstein, S., Zucker, C.L., and Fleiss, J.L., Some statistical methods useful in circulation research, *Circ. Res.*, 47, 1, 1980.

11. Zar, J.H., *Biostatistical Analysis*, Prentice Hall, New Jersey, 1986, chap. 11.

12. Ludbrook, J., Advantages of permutation (randomization) tests in clinical and experimental pharmacology and physiology, *Clin. Exp. Pharmacol. Physiol.*, 21, 673, 1994.

13. Krebs, H.A. and Henseleit, K., Untersuchungen über die Harnestoffbildung im Tierkorper, *Hoppe-Seyler's Zeit. Physiol. Chem.*, 210, 33, 1932.

14. Blinks, J.R., Method for study of contraction of isolated heart muscle under various physical conditions, *Circ. Res.*, 9, 342, 1961.

15. Doring, H.J. and Dehnert, H., *The Isolated Perfused Warm Blooded Heart According to Langendorff*, Biomesstechnik-Verlag, 40, March 1988.

16. Winslow, R.M., *Hemoglobin-based Red Cell Substitutes*, Johns Hopkins University Press, Baltimore, 1992, chap. 6.

17. Neely, J.R., Liebermeister, H., Battersby, E.J., and Morgan, H.E., Effect of pressure development on oxygen consumption by isolated rat heart, *Am. J. Physiol.*, 212, 804, 1967.

18. Lockwood, A.P.M., Ringer solutions and some notes on the physiological basis of their ionic composition, *Comp. Biochem. Physiol.*, 2, 241, 1961.

19. Hubbard, J.I., Llinas, R., and Quastel, D.M.J., *Electrophysiological Analysis of Synaptic Transmission*, Edward Arnold, London, 1969, chap. 8.

20. Krebs, H.A., Body size and tissue respiration, *Biochim. Biophys. Acta*, 4, 249, 1950.

21. Inoue, F., MacLeod, B.A., and Walker, M.J.A., Intracellular potential changes following coronary occlusion in isolated perfused rat hearts, *Can. J. Physiol. Pharmacol.*, 62, 658, 1984.

22. Geddes, L.A., Subintegumental electrodes, in *Electrodes and the Measurement of Bioelectric Events*, Wiley-Interscience, New York, 1973, chap. 3.

23. Beckman, K.J. and Hariman, R.J., Extracellular recording techniques, in *Electrophysiology and Pharmacology of the Heart*, Dangman, K.H. and Miura, D.S. Eds., Marcel Dekker, New York, 1991, chap. 4.

24. Dresdner, K.P., Standard and ion-selective microelectrodes, in *Electrophysiology and Pharmacology of the Heart*, Dangman, K.H. and Miura, D.S. Eds., Marcel Dekker, New York, 1991, chap. 2.

25. Goldstein, N.N. and Free, M.J., *Foundations of Physiological Instrumentation*, Charles C. Thomas, Springfield, IL, 1979, chap. 3.

26. Sinnaeve, A. and Tassignon, H., Signal Averaged ECG, technical principles, possibilities and limitations, in *Cardiac Pacing and Electrophysiology: A Bridge to the 21st Century*, Aubert, A.E., Ector, H., and Stroobandt, R., Eds., Kluwer Academic Publishers, Dordrecht, 1994, chap. 11.

27. Bezanilla, F., A high capacity data recording device based on a digital audio processor and a video cassette recorder, *Biophys. J.*, 47, 437, 1985.

28. Furukawa, Y., Akahane, K., Ogiwara, Y., and Chiba, S., K^+ channel blocking and anti-muscarinic effects of a novel piperazine derivative, INO 2628, on the isolated dog atrium, *Eur. J. Pharmacol.*, 193, 217, 1991.

Chapter 5

In Vivo Cardiac Measurements in the Conscious Rat

Tony Hebden

Contents

1. Introduction

In simple terms, the function of the heart is to ensure that blood flow within the vasculature is maintained. This is achieved by the myocardium imparting energy to the blood, a process which occurs because the heart is able to contract. Since contractility is the key to the function of the heart, it is not altogether surprising that the most measured variable in cardiac research is pressure and rate of change of pressure ($\pm dP/dt$). Measurement of intracardiac pressures provides valuable insight into the functional status of the heart. For example, an elevation in left ventricular end diastolic pressure or a reduction in left ventricular end systolic pressure are both indicative of an impairment in left ventricular function such as is seen following an acute myocardial infarction or in congestive heart failure.

Since the heart is a pump, to obtain a more quantitative picture of cardiac performance, cardiac output should also be measured. For example, following an experimental acute myocardial infarction, it is possible for left ventricular end diastolic pressure to increase while cardiac output is maintained by compensatory mechanisms. However, it is also possible to see a large fall in cardiac output along with an increase in left ventricular end diastolic pressure during experimental acute myocardial infarction. Clearly then, it is also important to monitor cardiac output along with intracardiac pressures when performing cardiac research. Measuring cardiac output is of particular value in chronic heart disease, as it is a primary indicator of the stage of the disease. That is, as the disease progresses, cardiac output will progressively fall. Indeed, cardiac index, which is cardiac output divided by surface area, is one of the main parameters used to determine whether a patient requires cardiac transplantation.

By monitoring pressure profiles within the chambers of the intact heart as well as cardiac output, the investigator is able to quantify cardiac function under physiological and pathophysiological conditions such as experimental acute myocardial infarction and in response to interventions such as administration of an inotropic agent or aortic constriction. Techniques for measuring intracardiac pressures and cardiac output in conscious, freely moving rats are described below.

1.1. Application of the *In Vivo* Preparation

Typically, *in vivo* cardiac experiments are more time consuming and costly than *in vitro* cardiac experiments. Furthermore, because of the morbidity and mortality associated with *in vivo* experimentation, as well as the fact that investigators are usually limited to using one or two animals per day, it can take several weeks to complete a study in which an *in vivo* preparation is utilized.

Despite these drawbacks, *in vivo* cardiovascular experimentation continues to be performed in laboratories throughout the world. The main reason that researchers use an *in vivo* preparation is because of its physiological validity. For example, it has been shown that the pressor response to vaso-pressin is diminished in conscious, freely moving rats with streptozotocin-induced diabetes mellitus.[1] However, pressor responsiveness to vasopressin was found to be normal in isolated arteries taken from rats with streptozotocin-induced diabetes mellitus.[2] The most likely reason for this disparity is that the *in vitro* studies involved looking at the responsiveness of large conduit vessels, while the responses observed *in vivo* reflected changes in the true resistance vessels, namely, the arterioles. The concept of physiological validity can also be applied to myocardial tissue. For example, an isolated heart is not innervated and the pericardium has been removed. Furthermore, an isolated working heart is usually pumping Kreb's solution (or a facsimile thereof). Not only is such a solution less viscous than whole blood and therefore requires less work to pump, but it is devoid of a number of its constituents such as red blood cells, platelets, white blood cells, hormones, and lipids.

Whether such disparities ultimately make a difference to the results obtained is open to debate. However, if the goal of the researcher is to extrap-olate the experimental data to the healthy conscious whole animal or even the clinical setting, then it is logical to use a model that approximates that condition as closely as possible.

2. Measuring Pressure

2.1. Pressure Monitoring System

In order to measure pressure and rate of change of pressure within the heart, three pieces of equipment are required:

1. *Pressure transducer.* There are a number of excellent discussions on these elsewhere to which the reader is referred.[3,4] Probably the most popular model used for this type of experiment is the Gould Statham transducer (Gould Instrument Systems, Inc., Valley View, OH).

2. *Catheter.* This allows the investigator to directly access the chamber or blood vessel she/he wishes to record from. Catheters, which are usually made of plastic, can typically be divided into two types: (a) the fluid-filled catheter and (b) the catheter-tip transducer. The latter is basically a pressure transducer that is small enough to fit on the tip of an intra-vascular catheter. Hence it is not fluid filled and connects directly to an amplifying circuit rather than a pressure transducer as is the case with the fluid-filled catheter.

3. *Recording device.* This converts the signal generated by the transducer into a trace that can be viewed and/or recorded. The best recording

devices currently available are the Thermal array recorders manufactured by Gould Instruments Systems Inc.

To accurately record a pressure profile requires a system with acceptable frequency characteristics. In an excellent review of the literature, Geddes[3] concluded that to adequately reproduce a blood pressure wave requires a monitoring system that possesses a uniform sinusoidal frequency response to at least the fifth harmonic, since five harmonics represents at least 98% of the variance. That is, the monitoring system should not underdamp or overdamp the pressure signal up to five times the frequency of the signal. For example, for rats with a heart rate of 360 beats/min or 6 Hz, the monitoring system (from the tip of the catheter in the vessel to the pen recording the trace on the recorder paper) should have give a flat frequency response to at least 30 Hz (5×6 Hz). Determining the frequency response characteristics for a particular system is described in Section 2.1.1.

With a catheter-tip transducer, the transducer is positioned directly into the blood vessel or cardiac chamber. Therefore, there will be no damping of the signal engendered by the pressure wave having to travel down a column of fluid, as is the case with a fluid-filled catheter. The most popular catheter-tip transducers produced commercially are manufactured by Millar Instruments Inc. of Houston, TX. These have been shown to have a flat frequency to at least 2000 Hz, which is well beyond what is required to accurately measure pressure waves *in vivo*.

Despite the outstanding frequency response of the Millar catheter, a number of researchers still prefer to use fluid-filled catheters as they afford several advantages:

1. They are relatively inexpensive, whereas catheter-tip transducers are very expensive.
2. Catheter-tip transducers have a limited lifespan, mainly because they are quite delicate.
3. Once the tip of the catheter is in place it is not possible to re-calibrate the transducer since it is physically in the vessel or chamber. Therefore, it is necessary to calibrate the transducer before and after the experiment and assume that any drift is linear.

There is the option of electronic calibration with this equipment, but it is always advisable to perform a manual calibration with a mercury manometer to guarantee the accuracy of the electronic calibration. With the fluid-filled system the transducer is outside the animal, and thus calibration of the transducer can be done repeatedly.

There is good experimental evidence to show that a fluid-filled catheter can be designed that will give a flat frequency response up to and beyond the fifth harmonic. In 1980 Gardiner et al.[5] obtained a flat frequency response to at least 35 Hz, using a catheter constructed from 80 cm of PE50 polyethylene tubing (internal diameter of 0.58 mm) joined to a 7 cm length of PE10 tubing (internal diameter of 0.28 mm). Making such a catheter is straightforward. The two pieces of tubing are heat-welded together over a low flame, the patency of the lumen being maintained by introduction of a thin piece of wire prior to melting the tubing together. The patency of the bond is maintained using epoxy resin. It is worth noting that the PE10 tip is narrow enough to be introduced into almost any artery or cardiac chamber of even very small animals.

We have shown that a fluid-filled catheter can also be used to accurately monitor left ventricular pressure and rate of change of left ventricular pressure in conscious, freely moving rats.[6] The catheter was almost identical to that of Gardiner et al.,[5] except that the PE50 tubing was slightly longer at 100 cm.

2.1.1. Determining the damping characteristics and frequency response of the pressure monitoring system

The simplest test of the damping characteristics of a catheter system is called the "transient method" or the method of Warburg.[7] The catheter tip is subjected to an instantaneous pressure increase and the decay of the signal is then used to calculate the natural frequency of the system as well as the damping ratio. The calculations necessary to determine these values are outlined in the paper by Warburg.[7]

Measuring the frequency response of the system is a little more complex. The best method is called the "sinusoidal method" and involves measuring the output signal when the input signal is of known frequency and fixed amplitude. The reader is referred elsewhere[5,8] for a detailed description of the equipment and methodology.

Making the above measurements is very time-consuming and therefore cannot be performed prior to each experiment. One way to obtain a measure of the damping of a pressure monitoring system that is already in place is to look for the inflection in the arterial pressure trace caused by the closure of the aortic valve (the dichrotic notch). If it is present, then the system is not overdamped. However, it is a somewhat crude measurement, as it will be present in an underdamped system.

2.2. Catheter Implantation

The acute, conscious model is a closed chest preparation, which means that catheters cannot be introduced directly into the heart as they are with an open chest preparation.

Procedure

1. The animal is anesthetized by intraperitoneal (IP) injection of the short-acting barbiturate sodium methohexital (60 mg/kg) (Brietal sodium, Eli Lilly, Toronto). The animal will remain unconscious for approximately 20 min so it is advisable to have a bolus dose of the anesthetic prepared for injection. Note that when the anesthetic begins to wear off the animal will regain consciousness very rapidly; therefore, it is advisable to continually test the level of consciousness of the animal throughout the procedure. The simplest way to do this is to pinch the skin between the toes of the hind feet to see if a withdrawal reflex is present.

2. Once the animal is anesthetized, it is necessary to isolate the blood vessels associated with catheter implantation. If measuring pressure in the left ventricle, the left common carotid artery is isolated, while for the right atrium or right ventricle the right jugular vein is isolated. If the experiment involves administration of drugs into the vascular system, a jugular vein should also be isolated so that one can implant one or more small PE10 polyethylene catheters. Whichever vessel is isolated, the technique is basically the same and is described below:

3. With the rat lying on its back, the fur on the underside of the neck is shaved using animal clippers.

4. A 1- to 2-cm incision is then made in the skin of the neck directly above the jugular vein and carotid artery. These vessels are easily located, as one can see the pressure waves transmitted from them. A scalpel can be used, but a small pair of surgical scissors (Fine Science Tools, Vancouver, BC) is preferred as this reduces the risk of cutting through the jugular vein, which lies close to the skin surface.

Note: *Remember, when using scissors, always keep the tips pointing upward.*

5. To isolate the blood vessels, blunt dissect the connective tissue, fat, and, in the case of the carotid artery, the muscle in which the vessels are lying. To do this, a pair of blunt-tipped surgical scissors is required (Fine Science Tools). The preferred technique is to close the scissors, push them into the connective tissue, muscle, or fat and then slowly open them. This procedure is repeated until the vessels are visible. The vessels are usually encased in a thin layer of adipose tissue that needs to be removed prior to cannulation of the vessel.

Note: **Do not** *attempt to remove the layer of adipose tissue with scissors as blood vessels are easily damaged.*

6.   The next step involves preparing a route for exteriorization of the catheter. For this, a hollow metal tube called a trochar is required. This is made by cutting a 6 to 8 cm length of hollow metal tubing (approximately 2 to 3 mm in diameter) and making it sharp at one end (Figure 1). This is achieved by cutting one end of the tubing at an angle of approximately 45° or by rubbing it at a 45° angle against sandpaper. The sharpened end of the trochar is introduced into the incision and is pushed **subcutaneously around the side of the neck** and exteriorized at the nape of the neck. If the skin in that area is too tough for the sharpened end of the trochar to penetrate, then a small incision can be made with a scalpel blade at the nape of the neck and the tip of the trochar pushed through. The catheter is then fed backward through the trochar until approximately 10 cm of the catheter tip projects from the initial incision (Figure 2A).

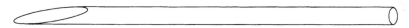

Figure 1
The trochar is approximately 6 to 8 cm in length, with an internal diameter of about 2 to 3 mm.

7.   The trochar is now pulled backward over the catheter, leaving approximately 10 cm of the catheter projecting from the ventral incision, while the rest of the catheter is tunneled sub-cutaneously and exteriorized at the nape of the neck (Figure 2B).

8.   To the end of the catheter projecting from the nape of the neck is attached a 5-ml hypodermic syringe containing 3 to 4 ml 0.9% saline with 12.5 U/ml heparin. The catheter is flushed with 1 to 2 ml of this solution, care being taken to ensure that no air is trapped in it.

9.   Prior to catheterization, the blood vessel must be cleaned of connective tissue and fat. To achieve this, two pairs of Graefe forceps are used (Fine Science Tools). One pair of forceps is slipped underneath the vessel in order to lift it up and so make it easier to access. With the second pair of forceps in the other hand, the connective tissue and fat is peeled off the vessel. The tissue will come away from the artery or vein very easily.

Note: *Do not pull or tug the vessel too much as it can either split or spasm, either of which can be a major problem. This step is necessary as it is important to have a clear, unobstructed section of blood vessel (5 mm to 1 cm in length). It is possible to cannulate a vessel with this tissue still attached, but this is not recommended.*

10.   The next step involves inserting the catheter into the jugular vein or carotid artery. In either case, the technique is the same:

11.   Slip the curved tips of a pair of Graefe forceps underneath the vessel; then open the forceps so that there is no blood flow in the vessel between

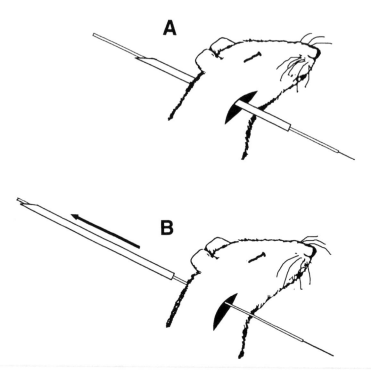

Figure 2
(A) The sharp end of the trochar is introduced into the ventral incision and tunneled sub-cutaneously to the neck, where it is exteriorized. The PE50/PE10 catheter is then fed backward up the trochar. (B) The trochar is pulled backward over the catheter (in the direction of the arrow), leaving the catheter in position.

the tips. It may prove necessary to use some modeling clay to hold the forceps in place, as both hands have to be free in order to cannulate the vessel (Figure 3A).

12.   Tie two ligatures using 3-0 silk suture proximally and distally to where the vessel is to be cut (Figure 3B) as these will be used to anchor the catheter once it is in place. Note that the proximal tie (i.e., that at the head end of the vessel) should be tied tightly while the other should be loose.

13.   Using a pair of extra fine curved iris scissors (Fine Science Tools), make a single cut into the vessel midway between the tips of the Graefe forceps. This cut should be no more than 50% of the thickness of the vessel so that the lumen is exposed. The best way to achieve the accuracy required is to lean forward and to one side of the animal so that one's eyes are at the same level as the blood vessel. By looking from the side at this level it becomes easier to see how deep one is cutting into the vessel. If the cut is not deep enough, it will be very difficult to introduce the tip of the catheter into the lumen; if it is too deep there is the risk of tearing the vessel in two when attempting to introduce the catheter.

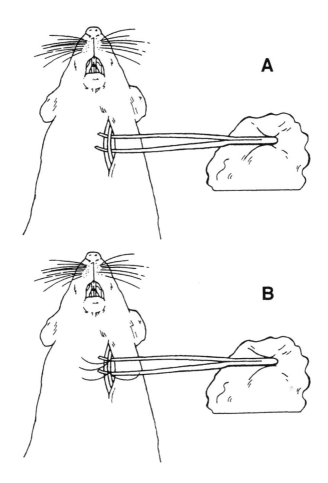

Figure 3

(**A**) Blood flow is stopped by the placement of Graefe forceps underneath the blood vessel. Note that modeling clay can be used to hold the forceps in place. (For clarity, the pressure catheter is not shown.) (**B**) Prior to cannulation, silk sutures are placed around the vessel. Note that the proximal ligature is tied tightly, while the distal ligature is loosely tied. (For clarity, the pressure catheter is not shown.)

This is why it is essential that there be a clear section of vessel to work with that is free of connective tissue and fat.

14. Since the tip of the catheter (PE10 tubing) is approximately the same diameter or even bigger than the lumen of the vessel, it is necessary to temporarily widen the exposed lumen in order to introduce the catheter tip. To do this requires Dumont #7 curved forceps ("watchmaker's" forceps) (Fine Science Tools). Holding these in the right hand, the closed tips of the forceps are inserted approximately 1 to 2 mm into the lumen of the vessel and then opened slightly to widen the lumen (Figure 4).

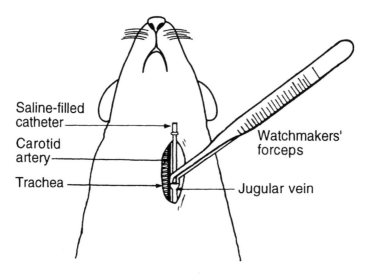

Saline-filled catheter

Carotid artery

Trachea

Watchmakers' forceps

Jugular vein

Figure 4
Implantation of a catheter in the jugular vein of the rat. Watchmaker forceps, held in one hand, are used to widen the lumen of the cut vessel, while the tip of the PE10 catheter is introduced into the vessel with the other hand. Note that the carotid artery lies more deeply than the vein and is located alongside the trachea. The artery is buried in muscle and therefore blunt dissection is required in order to view it. (Ligatures are not shown for clarity.)

15. The pressure-monitoring catheter is flushed with heparinized saline with the left hand, then the tip of the catheter is grasped between thumb and index finger of the left hand and guided between the tips of the forceps into the open lumen of the vessel (Figure 4). Once in the lumen, the Dumont forceps can be removed.

16. The catheter is fed down the vessel until it abuts against the lower arm of the Graefe forceps. The forceps need to be removed for cannulation to continue. This is not a problem with a jugular vein cannulation: one simply removes them and the modeling clay. However, more care is required if cannulating an artery because removing the forceps will allow blood to be pumped up the artery, and this can potentially blow the catheter out of the lumen and also cause significant blood loss. One way to resolve this is to loosely tie the catheter into the artery with the distal ligature (i.e., the one nearer the heart) so that it is held in place, then with the left hand hold the vessel up by the free ends of the suture and with the right hand push the catheter approximately 1 cm further into the vessel so that the tip is now in the thoracic cavity. At this point one no longer needs to pull up on the ligature as the carotid artery is suffi- ciently filled by the catheter that blood pressure will no longer be able to push it out. The Graefe forceps can now be removed from underneath the vessel.

17. The free (PE50) end of the catheter is now disconnected from the 5-ml syringe and connected to a pressure transducer. The preferred dome for

the transducer is described in detail elsewhere[9] and so will not be discussed here.

18. Using two pairs of curved Graefe forceps, the catheter is now advanced slowly down the vessel. The technique for this is that the investigator holds onto the distal knot with one pair of forceps and gently pushes the catheter into the vessel approximately 2 to 3 mm at a time with the other pair.

19. While implanting the catheter, the investigator should be watching the pressure trace on the recorder. The latter is critical for placement, since it is only possible to know that the catheter is in place when the correct pressure trace is observed. For example, one knows that the catheter tip has gone from the ascending aorta into the left ventricle when the pulse pressure (systolic pressure–diastolic pressure) goes from the aortic value of approximately 50 mm Hg to the left ventricular value of approximately 120 mm Hg (Figure 5). Placement of the catheter can be tricky, and, if it is clear that it has missed the intended target, then the catheter should be pulled back several centimeters and the investigator should try again.

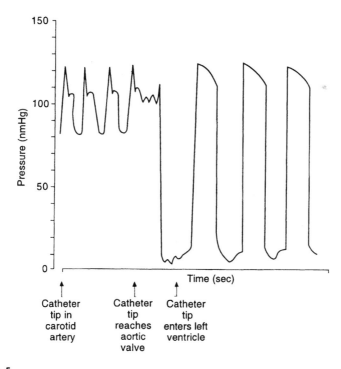

Figure 5

Typical pressure trace showing the tip of the catheter being advanced from the ascending aorta into the left ventricle. The change in the pressure profile is very obvious.

20.   When the catheter is correctly positioned it needs to be anchored firmly into place. This is achieved by tying both ligatures tightly around the vessel and catheter. Tygon is not prone to collapsing under pressure so the ligatures can be tied tightly. Using a third ligature is of value to ensure that the catheter (and hence its tip) does not move when the animal regains consciousness and begins to move around the cage, groom itself, and so forth.

21.   The wound site is now irrigated with 0.9% saline and dried with gauze (it is usually clean, with little blood being present) and the ventral incision closed using 7.5 mm Michel suture clips (Fine Science Tools).

22.   In order to allow the rat free movement, but at the same time protect the catheter(s) exteriorized at the nape of the neck, it is necessary to place the animal in a harness. The harness is easily made and can be one of many different designs. Probably the easiest is to make it so that it looks like a waistcoat. That is, it has two holes for the front legs to pass through and Velcro stitched on either side of the front so that it can be closed along the ventral surface of the animal (Figure 6). Glued to the dorsal surface of the harness is a Perspex block to which is secured a thin wire spring (diameter approximately 3 mm).

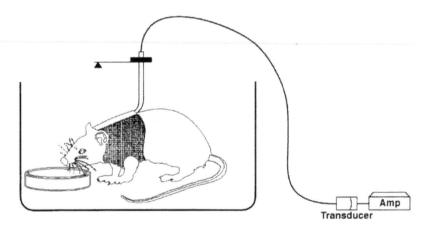

Figure 6

Diagram showing animal in tethered harness in cage following surgery. Note the spring connected to the universal swivel that protects the catheter from being chewed by the animal. (Figure used with the kind permission of Dr Terry Bennett, University of Nottingham.)

23.   The PE50 end of the catheter is removed from the transducer dome, heat sealed, and then fed through a hole in the harness and Perspex block. Finally, it is pushed up the length of the thin wire spring and reconnected to the transducer dome.

24.   The end of the spring is tethered to a counter-balanced support which allows the animal free movement in the cage in which it is placed (Figure 6). A water bowl should be placed in the cage after the animal wakes

up from surgery as they are usually thirsty. Whether one wishes to have water and/or food in the cage prior to, or even during, the experiment is left to the discretion of the investigator.

25.   Following 5 hours of recovery from anesthesia, the experiment can begin.

2.3.   Important Considerations

When working with a fluid-filled catheter system it is essential that all bubbles be removed from the fluid within the system as air is compressible and so will dampen any signal by lowering the natural frequency of the system. One way to do this is to boil the saline for several minutes prior to its introduction into the monitoring system. This process, which is called degassing, ensures that bubble formation in the saline during the experiment will be minimal.

Implanted catheters are in direct contact with blood and therefore, as a foreign surface, are prone to having clots form upon them. If one forms over the tip of the catheter or in the lumen of the catheter, the signal can become damped or even lost. To reduce the possibility of this occurring, the catheters should be flushed with degassed saline at least once per hour. In order to prevent clot formation, heparinized, degassed saline should be used to fill the system and flush the catheters. A concentration of 12.5 U/ml has been found to work very well, since this appears to prevent clot formation without overtly compromising the hemostatic mechanism.

Finally, the transducer should always be kept at the level of the heart of the animal being investigated. This will remove any anomalous effects caused by hydrostatic pressure.

3.   Measuring Flow

Techniques used to measure cardiac output can be divided into two categories: microspheres and flow probes.

3.1.   Microspheres

Microspheres are very easy to use, and the principle behind their use is extremely straightforward. They are plastic spheres with a diameter slightly greater than that of a capillary, and thus when injected into the cardiovascular system will lodge in the capillary beds in numbers which will be proportional to the flow to that bed.

This is a simple, reliable method that can produce excellent data. However, the major criticism with using microspheres to measure cardiac output or regional flows is that one is seeing flow "snapshots." That is, one is only seeing flow for the time when the microspheres were injected. Thus, it is not possible to get continuous flow measurements during an experiment. Furthermore, the investigator has to wait until the experiment is completed to obtain the flow data. Thus, if it is clear that the flow data are not correct at a certain time (e.g., the control period) then the data from the experiment may well have to be scrapped, because by this point it is too late to repeat the microsphere injection.

3.2. Flow Probes

Because of the above problems, many researchers prefer to measure cardiac output using flow probes. These can be divided into two categories, namely, electromagnetic and ultrasonic. Electromagnetic flow probes have been commercially available for a number of years. One of the most popular models is made by Skalar Medical (Litchfield, CT). The most commonly used type of electromagnetic probe is the perivascular flow probe. This is a rigid cuff that has an opening in it that allows it to be slipped over the vessel. Implantation of these probes is relatively easy as they come in a number of sizes so that they can be placed around almost any vessel.

There are two types of ultrasonic probe commonly in use: One type measures the transit time of ultrasound waves projected into the bloodstream ("transit-time method") and is manufactured by Transonics Systems Inc. (Ithaca, NY). The second type of flow probe measures Doppler shift within the blood stream ("Doppler method"). Like the electromagnetic flow probes, the ultrasonic probes come in a variety of sizes so that they can be placed around almost any blood vessel.

3.3. Implantation of a Flow Probe

Irrespective of which flow probe is chosen to measure ascending aortic blood flow, the surgical technique is the same and is described here. The technique described for implantation is based upon the method of Smith and Hutchins[10] as modified by Smits et al.[11]

Note: *Any experiment involving the implantation of a flow probe in the thoracic cavity of a rat and the subsequent measurement of blood flow in the conscious state is a chronic study, as the animal needs to recover for at least 3 to 4 days following surgery.*

Procedure

1.   For a 300-g rat an electromagnetic flow sensor or Doppler shift sensor with a diameter in the range of 2.5 to 3 mm should be chosen. A snug fit is preferable when placing either of these sensors, because it has been found that in order to gather accurate flow data, the cuff needs to fit

tightly. However, this is not essential in chronic studies, because any gap between the sensor and vessel will rapidly become infiltrated within 3 to 4 days following surgery. With the transit-time flow probes one should use a 2.5S or 3S sensor (Transonic Systems Inc.). By their design, these flow sensors will have a gap between the aorta and the reflecting plate of the probe when implanted. Again, however, the signal will be restored over 3 to 4 days as infiltration of the space occurs.

2. Autoclave all instruments and sterilize the flow probe with ethylene oxide. Prior to surgery put the probe in sterilized saline. For surgery wear a surgical mask and gloves. These steps should remove the need to treat the animal with antibiotics, although it is advised that following surgery a single intramuscular injection of 7 mg/kg ampicillin (Bristol-Myers Squibb, Montreal) be given.

3. The rat is anesthetized by IP injection of 60 mg/kg pentobarbital sodium (Abbott Laboratories Ltd., Montreal).

4. It is then placed on its back and with a pair of animal clippers the chest, including the area around the right armpit, is shaved. This should then be swabbed with betadine scrub (Purdue Frederick Inc., Pickering, ON).

5. Since this is an open-chest operation, the rat must be intubated. To do this it is essential to first ensure that the mouth stays open. One approach is to pull the upper jaw open by securing it with a rubber band (Figure 7). The tongue is then lifted upward with one hand (remember that the rat is on its back), and the tip of a PE240 cannula is inserted carefully past the vocal cords into the trachea. The investigator needs to be able to see the vocal cords prior to attempting intubation. This is done by shining a bright light over the shaved neck of the animal and looking directly down the throat while holding its tongue upward.

6. The free end of the cannula is attached to a Harvard small animal respirator (Harvard Instruments, South Natick, MA), which is then switched on at a setting of 60 breaths/min with a tidal volume of 2.5 to 3 ml. If the chest wall moves in time with the respirator, then the animal has been successfully intubated. The respirator can now be switched off until it is needed. If the abdominal wall of the animal moves instead, then the investigator has cannulated the stomach and the cannula must then be removed and another attempt made at intubation.

7. Make a 1- to 2-mm incision in the skin above the sixth right intercostal space, using small dissecting scissors or a scalpel (Fine Science Tools). Using blunt-tipped dissecting scissors, separate the skin from the muscle. Then create a purse-string suture around the dissected incision. This suture should not be pulled tight.

8. Make an incision in the skin above the third right intercostal space from the center of the sternum to where the right foreleg meets the trunk.

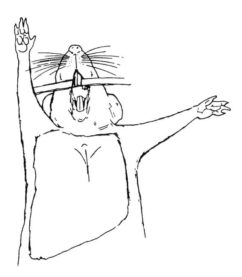

Figure 7
Anesthetized animal immediately prior to intubation. Note the placement of the rubber band underneath the upper teeth to hold the mouth open and also the positioning of the forelegs. The latter makes it easier to perform a thoracotomy.

9.   Using blunt-tipped dissecting scissors, separate the pectoral muscle from the underlying tissue. Once this is done cut through it cleanly with a pair of sharp scissors.

10. Using blunt-tipped dissecting scissors, dissect the rectus abdominus muscle free from the underlying tissue. It is attached to the sternum by a tendon at the third intercostal space. Cut the muscle at the level of the tendon.

11. The investigator can now perform a thoracotomy. Before doing this, the respirator should be started on a setting of 60 to 70 breaths/min at a tidal volume of 3 ml.

12. Using Graefe serrated eye dressing forceps (Fine Science Tools), blunt dissect **with extreme care** a small hole through the intercostal muscle approximately 5 mm from the sternum in the third intercostal space. Into this hole insert the tips of a pair of Moria fine forceps with 45° tips (Fine Science Tools) and use them to lift the thoracic wall upward. Using a pair of blunt-tipped dissecting scissors, cut through the intercostal muscle and pleural membranes for a distance of approximately 15 mm along the intercostal space. Be very careful when doing this, as it is easy to pierce the right lung.

13. Cut a small piece of sterile gauze and wet it in sterile 0.9% saline. Place this in the thoracic cavity and, with the aid of a pair of curved Graefe forceps, use it to move the lung out of the surgical field.

14. Insert three sutures (Ethicon 3-0 silk) around the third and fourth ribs. The first suture should be at the edge of the incision furthest from the sternum. The second suture should be positioned toward the sternum approximately 5 mm from the first suture, and the third suture should be at the edge of the incision at the sternum. These sutures should not be tied (Figure 8). Note that the mammillary artery runs along the edge of the sternum directly beneath where the suture is placed; therefore be very careful when pushing the suture needle through the wall of the thorax.

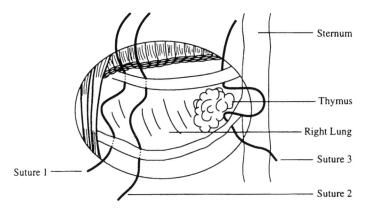

Figure 8
Placement of sutures following thoracotomy. (For clarity, the retractors are not shown.)

15. Insert a Goldstein or Agricola retractor (Fine Science Tools) into the incision and open it so that the contents of the right thoracic cavity are clearly visible.

16. At this point, the ascending aorta is usually not visible because it is covered by the thymus gland. Therefore, using a small pair of forceps, separate the portion of thymus impeding the approach to the aorta.

17. Remove any fat and connective tissue from the wall of the ascending aorta using small Graefe forceps. (Either curved or straight forceps can be used.) The aorta has a thick muscular wall and therefore is not easily penetrated by the blunt tips of forceps. However, with enough force it is possible to penetrate the aorta, so **be careful**. Remember, once the aorta is penetrated the experiment is over as the animal will die very rapidly.

18. Holding a 3-0 silk suture in the tips of a pair of Graefe curved forceps or curved Dumont #7 forceps (Fine Science Tools), pass the tips underneath the aorta. Using Dumont Forceps to do this is only possible if the tips have been blunted prior to experimentation, as the tips are very sharp and will easily pierce the aorta. Once the tips pass underneath to the other side of the aorta, grab the suture with a second pair of forceps and pull it partially through. Repeat this with a second length of suture so

that one now has two ligatures around the section of the aorta that has had the fat and connective tissue cleaned from it. These ligatures should be approximately 5 mm apart.

19. Using the curved Graefe forceps or blunted Dumont #7 forceps, gently blunt dissect the underside of the aorta so that the aorta between the ligatures is not attached to the wall of the thoracic cavity by connective tissue.

20. Approaching between the second and third chest sutures, place the aorta in the window of the flow sensor. Use the two sutures positioned around the aorta to place the aorta in the sensor.

21. When the aorta is in place, remove the sutures from around it. Then remove the gauze that was used to hold the right lung away from the aorta and finally remove the retractor.

22. To close the thorax, the three sutures around the third and fourth ribs must be tightly tied. The order for this is (1) pull and tie the second (middle) suture, (2) pull and tie the first suture (one furthest from the sternum), and finally (3) pull and tie the suture (the one closest to sternum).

23. Before cutting the loose ends of the suture, secure the sensor cable to the ribs using the first and second sutures. When this is completed the loose ends can be cut.

24. Using 5-0 surgical silk, repair the two muscles that were cut prior to the thoracotomy.

25. For the animal to breathe spontaneously, it is necessary to reintroduce a negative pressure into the thoracic cavity. Using blunt forceps, carefully stab a small hole in the sixth intercostal space at the site prepared prior to flow sensor placement. Insert a small silastic drainage tube which is connected to a vacuum pump and apply a vacuum of -10 cm H_2O to it. If the thorax has not been sealed correctly, it will not be possible to maintain a vacuum.

26. Switch off the respirator. The animal should breathe spontaneously at this point. If not, switch the respirator back on and check the sutures. If these are good then try increasing the CO_2 content of the inspired air and take the animal off the respirator again.

27. Suture the skin over the thoracotomy site but leave approximately 1 cm open.

28. Turn the rat onto its front and make an incision of approximately 2 cm between the shoulder blades. Blunt dissect subcutaneously from the incision to the inside of the right foreleg of the animal.

29. Pull the flow sensor cable under the skin from the thoracotomy site to the neck so that the cable connector is located in the neck.

30. Place two sutures in the muscle above the spinal cord at the incision site and tie the cable tightly to these sutures.

31. Suture the skin around the connector closed.

32. Close the 1-cm wound on the ventral surface that was left open to allow the sensor cable to be pulled subcutaneously and exteriorized at the nape of the neck.

33. Remove the endotracheal tube. In one movement, remove the drain from the chest and pull the purse-string suture so that the incision above it is closed.

34. The animal should recover for a minimum of 4 days before the experiment can be performed. On the morning of the experiment the animal has to be anesthetized (see Section 2.2) for intracardiac or intraarterial catheter implantation (if required) and so that the flow sensor connector can be attached to the lead, which is then fed via the harness and spring to the monitoring device (see Section 2.2 for details).

3.4. Limitations of Flow Probes

While either of the flow probes described above can be implanted around the ascending aorta to give a measure of cardiac ouput, they cannot be calibrated *in vivo*. Each system comes with electronic calibration, but a flow monitoring system should always be calibrated manually to ensure that the electronic calibration is accurate. It is possible to obtain a zero flow value by using a pneumatic occluder which is placed proximally to the flow probe and is used to occlude the blood vessel under investigation. However, in order to obtain a calibration line, a second value, which must be greater than zero flow, is required. One method is to leave the probe *in situ* after killing the animal at the end of the experiment and then to perfuse the vessel with blood. The accuracy of such a method must be questioned, however, as calibration is carried out in a preparation that is different from the one in which the experimental data was obtained. With the Doppler shift flow probes this problem can be resolved, at least in part, by quoting flow velocities as frequency changes[12] (Figure 9). This is acceptable, but the researcher has no measure of actual velocity.

4. Other Considerations

4.1. Conscious vs. Anesthetized Animals

General anesthetics, by their nature, have direct effects upon the central nervous system and consequently will almost certainly have effects on the cardiovascular system. For example, in rats it has been shown that the inhalant anesthetic halothane inhibits the sympathadrenal system;[13] in rabbits it causes vascular hyporesponsiveness to norepinephrine which persists up to 2 hours following recovery from anesthesia,[14] and in humans it has been found to depress cardiac baroreflex sensitivity in response to angiotensin II.[15]

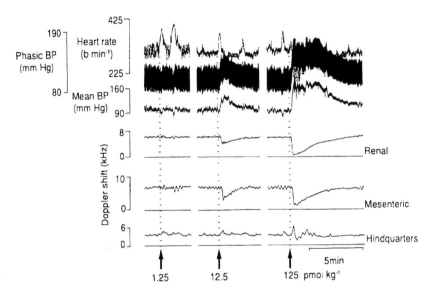

Figure 9

Typical data obtained from a conscious rat implanted with blood pressure catheter and Doppler shift ultrasonic flow probes. Note that flow is shown as a frequency shift. (Figure used with the kind permission of Dr. Terry Bennett, University of Nottingham.)

Pentobarbital sodium anesthesia has been shown to cause significant hypotension in dogs, a phenomenon not observed when animals were premedicated with fentanyl and anesthetized with alpha-chloralose.[16] This observation must be interpreted with caution, however, as Bennett and Gardiner[17] have shown that urethane-anesthetized rats maintain a normal blood pressure until challenged with a vasopressin antagonist, at which time they develop a profound hypotension. One interpretation of this finding is that since vasopressin was maintaining blood pressure, urethane was clearly inhibiting sympathoadrenal function. This observation is important, since it demonstrates that blood pressure cannot necessarily be used as an indicator of normal cardiovascular function.

It seems clear that the anesthetized preparation should be avoided whenever possible, since it is easy to question the validity of data obtained from such a preparation. While it is not always easy or even possible to perform conscious animal experiments, acute experiments using conscious small mammals such as rats are feasible. For example, it has been shown that there are no differences in cardiovascular status or in cardiac baroreflexes 5 h and 72 h after surgery performed on rats anesthetized with the short-acting barbiturate methohexitone sodium.[18] These results indicate that this barbiturate had no apparent carry over effects on cardiovascular function after 5 h of recovery from anesthesia. This is an important finding, since it demonstrates that it is possible to anesthetize a rat, implant catheters, allow the animal to recover for 5 h, and then perform the experiment all in one day.[5]

4.2. Adapting to Other Species

The techniques described above are not limited to the rat but can also be applied to larger animals such as pigs or dogs with minor modification, mainly because the anatomy of these animals is virtually identical, and thus it is simply a case of using larger flow probes, bigger surgical equipment such as retractors, more anesthetic, and so forth.

One advantage of using a larger animal is that typically more variables can be monitored. For example, it makes little sense to use rats when investigating regional myocardial blood flow following coronary artery occlusion, because the rat heart is simply too small to make valid measurements.

One disadvantage to using a larger animal is that the bigger the animal, the more expensive the experiment becomes as the cost and upkeep of the animal is greater, and the equipment required to perform the surgery tends to be larger and usually more elaborate. Probably the greatest disadvantage to using a large animal is not the expense, however, but rather the complexity associated with using a conscious preparation. Conscious *in vivo* experiments using large mammals are technically demanding, can be fraught with difficulty, and are simply not an option in a number of laboratories. Therefore, the majority of investigators who work upon large mammals in cardiac research use an acute, anesthetized preparation.

Acknowledgments

I would like to thank Dr. Terry Bennett, Department of Physiology and Pharmacology, University of Nottingham Medical School and Dr. Howard Nathan, Department of Cardiac Anaesthesia, University of Ottawa Heart Institute for their invaluable assistance in the preparation of this chapter.

References

1. Hebden, R. A., Bennett, T., and Gardiner, S. M., Pressor sensitivity to vasopressin, angiotensin II or methoxamine in diabetic rats, *Am. J. Physiol.*, 253, R726, 1987.
2. Hebden, R. A., Doroudian, A., and McNeill, J. H., Evidence for regionally selective changes in response to potassium chloride but not vasopressin or methoxamine in vasculature from diabetic rats, *Can. J. Physiol. Pharmacol.*, 66, 1464, 1988.
3. Geddes, L. A., *The Direct and Indirect Measurement of Blood Pressure*, Year Book Medical Publishers, Chicago, 1970.
4. Milnor, W. R., *Hemodynamics*, Waverley Press, Baltimore, 1982.

5. Gardiner, S. M., Bennett, T., and Kemp, P. A., Systemic arterial hypertension in rats exposed to short-term isolation; intra-arterial systolic and diastolic blood pressure and baroreflex sensitivity, *Med. Biol.*, 58, 232, 1980.

6. Schenk, J., Hebden, A., and McNeill, J. H., Measurement of cardiac left ventricular pressure in conscious rats using a fluid-filled catheter, *J. Pharm. Methods*, 27, 171, 1992.

7. Warburg, E., A method of determining the undamped natural frequency and the damping in overdamped and slightly underdamped systems of one degree of freedom by means of a square-wave impact, *Acta Physiol. Scand.*, 19, 344, 1949.

8. Ardill, B. L., Fentem, P. H., and Wellard, M. J., An electromagnetic pressure generator for testing the frequency response of transducers and catheter systems, *J. Physiol. (Lond)*, 192, 19P, 1967.

9. Ardill, B. L., Fentem, P. H., and Wellard, M. J., A design for the dome of a medical pressure transducer, *Bio-Med. Eng.*, 3, 160, 1968.

10. Smith, T. L. and Hutchins, P. M., Central hemodynamics in the developmental state of spontaneous hypertension in the unanesthetized rat, *Hypertension Dallas*, 1, 508, 1979.

11. Smits, J. F. M., Coleman, T. G., Smith, T. L., Kasbergen, C. M., Van Essen, H., and Struyker-Boudier, H. A. J., Antihypertensive effect of propranolol in conscious spontaneously hypertensive rats; central hemodynamics, plasma volume and renal function during beta-blockade with propranolol, *J. Cardiovasc. Pharmacol.*, 4, 903, 1982.

12. Gardiner, S. M., Compton, A. M., Bennett, T., and Hartley, C. J., Can pulsed Doppler technique measure changes in aortic blood flow in conscious rats?, *Am. J. Physiol.*, 259, H448, 1990.

13. Hoffman, W. E., Seals, C., Miletich, D. J., and Albrecht, R. F., Plasma and myocardial catecholamine levels in young and aged rats during halothane anesthesia, *Neurobiol. Aging*, 6, 117, 1985.

14. Spiss, C. K., Smith, C. M., Tsujimoto, G., Hoffman, B. B., and Maze, M., Prolonged hyporesponsiveness of vascular smooth muscle contraction after halothane anesthesia in rabbits, *Anesth. Analg.*, 64, 1, 1985.

15. Duke, P. C., Fownes, D., and Wade, J. G., Halothane depresses baroreflex control of heart rate in man, *Anesthesiology*, 46, 184, 1977.

16. Hebden, R. A. and Nathan, H. J., Effect of parathyroid hormone on myocardial blood flow and infarct size following coronary artery occlusion in the dog, *Can. J. Cardiol.*, 10, 477, 1994.

17. Bennett, T. and Gardiner, S. M., Hypotension following antagonism of the cardiovascular actions of vasopressin in urethane-anaesthetized Long Evans, Wistar and Sprague-Dawley rats, *J. Physiol. (Lond)*, 366, 51P, 1985.

18. Bennett, T. and Gardiner S. M., Cardiac baroreflex sensitivities to depressor stimuli following acute and chronic arterial catheterization in Long Evans and Brattleboro rats, *J. Physiol. (Lond)*, 372, 76P, 1986.

Chapter

The Isolated, Coronary-Perfused, Right Ventricular Wall Preparation

Thane G. Maddaford, Hamid Massaeli,
and Grant N. Pierce

Contents

0-8493-3332-6/97/$0.00+$.50
© 1997 by CRC Press, Inc.

1. Introduction

The isolated right ventricular wall, like the septal wall,[1] is a coronary-perfused cardiac muscle preparation which is composed of only a select portion of the whole heart. It is a relatively new technique[2-8] employed for the measurement of cardiac function, which offers distinct advantages over other more conventional techniques like the Langendorff (and its many variations) or superfused muscle preparations (like papillary or trabeculae muscles). It is the purpose of this treatise to discuss this technique, identify the advantages and limitations of this model, and describe its use in detail.

1.1. Advantages

It is important to emphasize the strengths and weaknesses associated with a technique, particularly when the methodology is relatively new. First and foremost, the right ventricular wall exhibits excellent tension development per gram of tissue weight. Maximal developed tension is ~60 g/g wet tissue weight, which is far better than most values of maximal tension development (5 to 15 g/g wet weight) in whole hearts perfused in a retrograde fashion.[9-13] The perfused interventricular septal muscle exhibits tension generation which is closer to the right ventricular wall (15 to 40 g/g wet weight).[14-15] The orientation of the muscle in the perfusion apparatus (consistently straight in one direction) may allow for a more efficient transfer of the force from the right ventricular wall to the recording transducer than occurs with the curving fiber orientation in the whole heart.

One obvious advantage of the perfused right ventricular wall in comparison to superfused muscles like the papillary is that it is perfused through the coronary arteries. This reduces the possibility of the tissue interior becoming hypoxic during the course of an experiment. Perfusion through the coronary artery also allows for the rapid delivery of a drug to the muscle, a feature which should be particularly appealing to pharmacologists. The delivery of compounds to the muscle is very fast for two reasons. First, because the tissue size is limited to just the right ventricle, there is limited vascular space and hence a reduction in the equilibration time. Second, a stopcock used to switch the perfusate solution to one which contains a drug is located in close proximity to the cannula (Figure 1). This allows for the drug to be rapidly introduced to the muscle and eliminates the time spent in the tubing itself prior to muscle

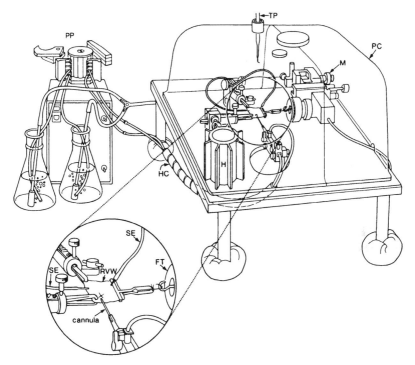

Figure 1

Perfused right ventricular wall experimental apparatus. RVW, coronary perfused right ventricular wall; FT, force transducer; SE, stimulating electrodes; PP, peristaltic pump; HC, perfusion line heating coil; TP, temperature probe to monitor chamber air temperature; H, heated water humidifier; M, micromanipulator for force transducer; PC, Plexiglas chamber cover. (From Meng, H. and Pierce, G.N., *J. Pharmacol. Exp. Ther.*, 256, 1094, 1991. With permission.)

perfusion. In the rabbit right ventricular wall, the exchange half-time for the vascular space is 5 s,[2] and this would likely be faster in the smaller rat muscle. Equilibration within the interstitial space is approximately 1 min in the rabbit right ventricular wall.[2] The rapid delivery of drugs into the coronary artery can be critical in ischemia/reperfusion studies, for example, which require an immediate delivery of drug to the muscle following ischemia.[3,4,6] The limited perfusion volume required for the right ventricular wall could also be beneficial when including expensive drugs or biological materials in the perfusate. The researcher using the right ventricular wall will require less of a drug at the conventional 1.5 ml/min flow rates than would be consumed in whole heart experiments with flow rates of 10 to 20 ml/min.[10-12]

In some cases, it is important to determine the function of the right ventricle in isolation if it is expected to be different than the left ventricle or the whole heart. For example, if the left ventricle suffers a myocardial infarction, the functional and structural responses of the left ventricle may be very different than the right ventricle. In such cases, study of the contractile characteristics of the right ventricular wall in isolation with the perfused right ventricular wall would be useful.

The right ventricular wall is more tolerant of ischemic insults than the whole heart. From a practical viewpoint, this tolerance is of great value during the cannulation and mounting of the muscle in the perfusion apparatus. It is not unusual, while setting up a heart in the perfusion apparatus, that relatively small time delays will occur before perfusion of the muscle is completely initiated. These delays in muscle perfusion can result in significant arrhythmias, contractile dysfunction, and cell damage in the heart before the researcher even begins an experiment. The capacity of the right ventricular wall to withstand small ischemic insults means that the researcher is under less pressure to initiate perfusion of the muscle immediately after removing the heart from the animal. This relative resistance to ischemia in the right ventricular wall also means that the time required to induce severe ischemic damage is greater in the right ventricular wall as opposed to the whole heart. For example, mild ischemic insult (~75% recovery of developed tension) requires a global ischemic duration of about 15 to 20 min in the whole heart and 30 min in the right ventricular wall. Severe ischemic damage (~10% recovery of developed tension) will occur after 30 min of no-flow perfusion in the whole heart vs. 75 min in the right ventricular wall. Thus, the researcher who wishes to examine mild, moderate, and severe ischemia has a window of only 10 to 15 min to use in the whole heart, as opposed to 45 min in the right ventricular wall. The short window will lead to experimental variability: a 1 min difference in the ischemic duration in the whole heart could result in a large difference in its recovery from ischemia. However, this longer duration will reduce the number of ischemic experiments that one can complete with the right ventricular wall in 1 day.

The right ventricular wall offers the investigator several important research opportunities not available to those using whole heart preparations. In some research applications, the investigator may not want the isotope or probe to mix in the volume of dead space found in the ventricular chamber. The measurement of ^{45}Ca flux in whole tissue is one example. The time it takes for the radioisotope to mix with the ventricular volume and the unknown intraventricular volume can create complications which make accurate measurements of the uptake of ^{45}Ca into the myocardial cells very difficult. The right ventricular wall does not have a ventricular cavity in which perfusate accumulates and therefore obviates this problem. It has been successfully employed in the past to monitor the uptake of ^{45}Ca (transsarcolemmal transport) into the myocardial cell.[2] This advantage could be potentially beneficial when using other probes where similar dilution or exchange problems exist.

A unique advantage of the right ventricular wall is the ability to continuously record electrical activity in this preparation. The whole heart is notorious for dislodging or damaging glass microelectrodes which are impaled into the beating muscle. Although the papillary muscle can be impaled and used to monitor electrical activity, these preparations are not ideal for ischemic experiments because they are superfused. Action potentials have been successfully recorded throughout ischemia and reperfusion in the right ventricular wall.[8,19] There appears to be no qualitative difference in the recordings obtained from papillary muscles and the right ventricular wall.[7] To our knowledge, the right ventricular wall remains as the best cardiac preparation from which to obtain electrical activity recordings in ischemic tissue.

A final advantage of the right ventricular wall preparation is theoretical at this point in time. The right ventricular wall is very thin. With a light placed under the muscle, it is very easy to see through the tissue and define gross structural features and vessel location. Because of this semitranslucent nature of the preparation, it may be ideal for use with fluorescent and photoactivated probes like fura-2 or other ion indicator probes. This is currently done with other muscle preparations[20] to monitor ion movements in the heart as it functions. The added benefit of the right ventricular wall over the superfused preparations is that the coronary vasculature is still intact. Of course, the apparatus described later in this chapter (and shown in Figure 1) would have to be modified substantially to accomodate a microscope and spectrofluorometry system capable of capturing the fluorescent signal.

1.2.   Disadvantages

It is also important to identify disadvantages associated with the use of this preparation. For the most part, we have found that the advantages outweigh the potential defects of the preparation. The most significant limitation of the preparation is that it does not contain all of the structural components of the whole heart. It is missing the left ventricle and the Purkinje fibers and other electrical conduction pathways present in a whole heart preparation. This is a shortcoming which also exists to varying degrees for the papillary and trabeculae muscles, and the interventricular septal preparation. For those interested in whole heart arrhythmogenesis, this may represent an important factor. It is also possible that data obtained in the right ventricle may not be applicable to the left ventricle or the heart as a whole. However, data obtained to date suggest that the general principles obtained in the right ventricle are similar to the left ventricle or the whole heart (i.e., a particular drug protects against ischemic insult; an inotropic intervention is effective, etc.).[3-8,16-18] Two other limitations of the right ventricular wall preparation are practical in nature. First, very small animals will have tiny hearts that will be very difficult to cannulate. Second, because there is less tissue available in a right ventricular wall as opposed to a whole heart, there will be less tissue available for subsequent biochemical assays or other experiments. There may not be, for example, sufficient starting tissue available for the investigator to isolate a viable membrane preparation. Several hearts must be pooled to obtain sufficient starting tissue.

2.   Materials and Methodology

2.1.   Equipment Needed

2.1.1.   Major electronic equipment

The Gilson Minipuls 2 multichannel peristaltic pump (Mandel Scientific Co. Ltd., Guelph, ON) is used to pump perfusate. The perfusate is heated by wrapping perfusion lines with silicone heating tape (11-463-58A, Fisher Scientific Ltd., Edmonton, AB). Temperature is controlled by an Electrothermal MC 228 temperature controller (11-463-46, Fisher Scientific Ltd.). Many other means of maintaining perfusate flow and temperature are currently available and acceptable. Temperature is monitored with a Sensortek digital thermometer (BAT- 8C, Bailey Instruments, Saddlebrook, NJ) using a thermocouple probe (H-08506-95, Cole-Parmer Instrument Co., Niles, IL). The heart is stimulated with a custom built stimulator (University of Manitoba). Isometric force generation is translated by a force transducer (FTD-0-100, Duram Instruments, Pickering, ON). Developed tension, resting tension and + and – dT/dt are recorded on a Linearcorder Mark VII chart recorder (WR3101 Western Graphtec, Irvine, CA). We have found this instrument to be very reliable over the years.

2.1.2.   Surgical instruments

All surgical instruments were purchased from Fine Science Tools, North Vancouver, BC. Micromosquito hemostats (13010-12), Dumont curved forceps (11272-14), and Moria straight blade spring scissors MC26/B (15372-62) are all important for the dissection and cannulation of the heart. Quality spring scissors are important since they allow for increased manual dexterity. The right ventricular wall is attached to the transducer by a special clamp made by modifying a 26-mm Schwartz microserrefine clamp (18052-01). Two 2 mm × 12 mm light gauge stainless steel strips are soldered to the ends of the clamp with nonlead solder.

2.1.3.   Custom built equipment and miscellaneous supplies

Adjustable tissue clamps are made by mounting 9-cm toothed forceps onto single drive manipulators. These in turn are mounted upon slotted adjustable Plexiglas supports. The force transducer is fixed to an X-Y-Z axis micromanipulator (25033-0, Fine Science Tools) to allow for adjustment of the heart in all planes. The manipulator is adjustable upon a vertical aluminum rod fixed to the Plexiglas stand. The stand is constructed of 40 cm × 40 cm × 2 cm thick Plexiglas sitting upon four 2 cm × 15 cm aluminum supports (Figure 1). Several strategically placed holes in the stand allow for waste perfusate efflux.

   In order to create a humid 37°C environment during experimental procedures of low or no flow ischemia, a heated water bath is installed and the stand covered with a Plexiglas hood. The hood is made of 5 mm thick Plexiglas and is 28 cm × 33 cm × 16 cm high. The heater is 5 cm wide by 20 cm deep and is regulated by a feedback-controlled unit built at the University of Manitoba.

Other miscellaneous supplies include: 6-0 C-1 suture needles with black braided silk, (Ethicon Ltd., Peterborough, ON), which is used to suture the cannula into the right coronary. Also, 5-0 braided silk A-52 (Ethicon Ltd.) is used to tie the clamp to the force transducer. The perfusion lines are made of Tygon R-3603 (AAC00004, Performance Plastic Corp., Akron, OH). Peristaltic pump manifold tubing is made by Elkay (LK116-0549-190, Elkay Products Inc., Shrewsbury, MA). The cannula is made with a 2-cm piece of Intramedic polyethylene tubing (7410, Becton Dickinson and Co., Parsippany, NJ) which has been flared on one end with heat. The cannula is then placed upon a 23 gauge G-1 syringe needle (5145, Becton Dickinson and Co., Rutherford, NJ) which fits snugly upon a Pharmaseal 3-way stopcock (K-75 Baxter Healthcare Corp., Valencia, CA).

2.2. Technique

Rats are anesthetized with a suitable anesthetic, sacrificed by decapitation, and then the heart is excised by cutting transversely across the ascending aorta, superior vena cava, and the pulmonary artery, 2 to 3 mm distal to the heart. The heart is then placed in a HEPES perfusate solution containing the following components (millimolar): NaCl, 140; KCl, 6; MgCl$_2$, 1; CaCl$_2$, 1; HEPES (*N*-[2-hydroxyethyl] piperazine-*N*´-[2-ethanesulfonic acid]), 6; and dextrose, 10; pH 7.4 at 20°C. We have used other conventional perfusion solutions (i.e., bicarbonate based) without adverse effects. Prior to the dissection of the heart, the peristaltic pump and heating apparatus should be turned on to allow for temperature stabilization at 37°C. The peristaltic pump has been previously calibrated and the temperature controller for the heating coil surrounding the perfusion lines is calibrated so that the perfusion solution entering the heart through the cannula is 37°C.

2.2.1. Dissection

The heart should be first placed on a dissection tray covered with a gauze sponge wet with the HEPES perfusate. The right and left atria are first dissected off, with care not to cut any of the large vessels entering or exiting the heart. The heart should be positioned with the right ventricle up, apex of the heart distal and vessels proximal.

The right ventricle should be removed as follows: the entire length of the cutting surface of one of the scissor blades is placed along the juncture of the right ventricle and septum so that one blade is entirely within the right ventricular cavity (Figure 2). The scissors are continually pushed further along the ventricle-septal border, while at the same time gently lifting the right ventricle to expose the endocardium and papillaries. Cutting is continued along the ventricle-septal border to within 2 mm of the aorta. Papillaries joining the

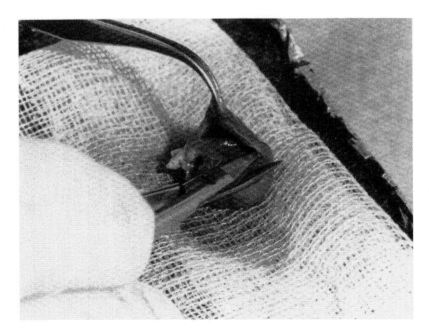

Figure 2
Photograph of the right ventricular wall being cut away from the septum.

ventricle to the septum were cut most proximal to the endocardial surface of the right ventricle. The scissors are positioned so that one of the cutting blades is within the ascending aorta and the other is in the middle of the left ventricle-septal space. A cut is made to sever the adjoining tissue. The right ventricle is oriented with the epicardial side upwards and is separated from the rest of the heart by cutting through the septum 2 mm below the point of origin of the coronaries in the aorta. The free right ventricular wall is oriented with the epicardial side down and aorta proximal. The coronaries are evident and the right ventricular wall should appear rectangular in shape. In this position, with the right coronary to the left side, an incision is made approximately 2 mm left of the opening of the vessel on the curled corner of the ventricular wall so it would lie horizontal in the dissection tray.

2.2.2. Cannulation

The right ventricular wall is pinned near the coronary with the endocardial side of the heart down and the coronaries proximal. The coronaries would appear as 1 mm openings in the aorta and approximately 2 to 4 mm apart. The head of the cannula is gently inserted 2 mm into the right coronary by adjusting the dissection tray and cannula, until a slight resistance is felt (Figure 3). The heart is successfully cannulated if the blood is cleared from the vessels of the heart. Perfusion flow rate is 1.5 ml/min. It is often helpful to guide the cannula with forceps while adjusting the dissection tray. Two obvious signs that the preparation is not receiving adequate perfusion are: (1) arrhythmias,

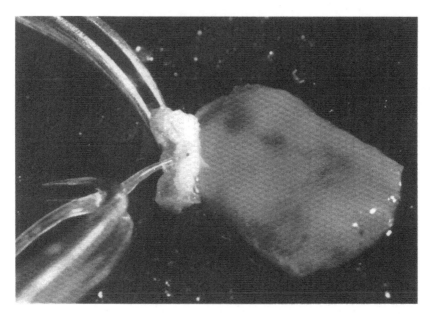

Figure 3
Photograph showing the cannula being inserted into the right coronary artery.

and (2) a dark red color of the muscle, indicating areas are not being cleared of blood.

The cannula must be sutured into the coronary in order to maintain constant perfusion to the heart. Suture silk (6-0) with a taper (C-1) needle is used because of the delicate work involved. The heart is braced by grasping the tissue near the coronary with the left hand. The suture needle is grasped with fine straight hemostats approximately 2 to 3 mm from the point of the needle. The tissue is impaled <1 mm right of the right coronary to a point which is below the bottom edge of the cannula and surrounding vessel. Slowly turning the hemostats clockwise (if using right hand), the curved needle would pass just under the vessel to the epicardial (upper) side of the ventricle until 1 to 2 mm of the needle tip is protruding (Figure 4). The needle is pulled through carefully, to a point at which only 3 cm of silk remains. The silk is trimmed equally on the other side. A single surgeon's knot is tied, using two sets of fine nonserrated curved tip forceps so that the loop is around the head of the cannula. Once secure, a double-loop surgeon's knot is tied carefully, being sure not to pull the cannula out of the vessel. The silk can be trimmed to within 1 mm of the knot.

There is a small bifurcating vessel running from the right coronary artery to the septum, which should be tied off to receive maximal perfusion to the right ventricular wall. The right wall is oriented with the endocardium dorsal. The small vessel is closed by tying a small loop of 5-0 silk around the small piece of septal tissue just above the cannula. It can also be clamped using a small microvascular serrefine.

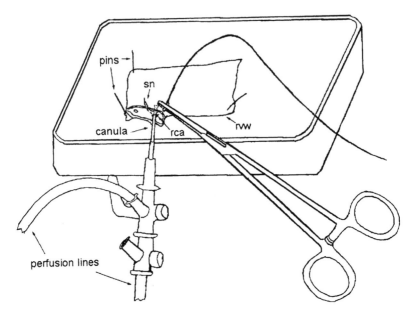

Figure 4
Illustration demonstrating the cannulation of the right coronary artery (rca) and insertion of the suture needle (sn) into the perfused right ventricular wall (rvw).

2.2.3. Mounting the right ventricle
The right ventricle, once securely cannulated, is clamped parallel to the orientation of the force transducer. Adjustable clamps attached to micromanipulators are used to first secure the most distal ends of the free wall. Micromanipulators are adjusted with sufficient tension so that the ventricle does not sag between the clamps. Care must be taken to clamp the ventricular tissue 1 to 2 mm left of the cannula without damaging the right coronary artery. Distal to the cannula, the ventricular wall is clamped on the peripheral edge, over its entire width, using a specially designed 12-mm wide microserrefine clamp (Figure 1). The clamp is attached to the force transducer with 5-0 silk. The horizontal force transducer rides on a micromanipulator to allow for vertical and horizontal adjustment. After the recording device has been turned on, resting tension should be increased to 2 to 3 grams. The stimulating electrodes are inserted at opposite ends of the heart as close as possible to the edge of the tissue.

2.2.4. Recording results
The heart is paced at 200 beats/min with a 9 millisecond duration at 200% of threshold voltage. The right ventricular wall is stretched in all horizontal planes, optimally, to maximize tension development. Developed tension is monitored while adjusting the heart in order to optimize stretch. The resting tension of the ventricle is gradually increased in 2- to 3-g increments by

carefully adjusting the transducer micromanipulator, followed by breaks of 5 min to allow for equilibration. An increase in resting tension is followed by an increase in developed tension. There is a slight drop in developed tension and resting tension shortly thereafter; however, there is always a net increase. Resting tension is increased to a point where developed tension is optimized. If it is increased beyond these optimal levels, developed force will decrease instead of increase. A general rule is to increase resting tension to a level of 5 g resting tension per 0.1 g of heart wet weight. Perfusate temperature should be maintained at 37°C, and can be monitored by inserting the temperature probe tip between the stopcock and perfusion line nearest the cannula. Hearts are allowed to equilibrate for at least 30 min with the perfusion apparatus uncovered before any experiments proceed.

2.3.   Representative Results

Typical recorded results for a perfused rat right ventricular wall preparation are depicted in Figure 5.

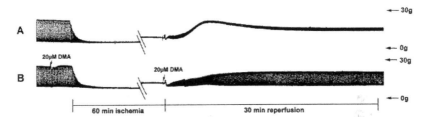

Figure 5
Representative recordings of tension development in two RVW (right ventricular wall) perfusion experiments. (**A**) Depicts tension in a RVW after control - 60 min ischemia followed by 30 min of reperfusion. (**B**) Depicts tension in a RVW perfused for 3 min with 20 μM DMA (5-[N,N-dimethyl]-amiloride), followed by a 60 min ischemia. DMA (20 μM) was also included in the first 3 min of the 30 min reperfusion period.

2.4.   Potential Problems and Remedies

Due to the size of the heart and the nature of the dissection, there can be difficulties with this preparation. With inexperience, it is easy to damage important vessels and render the heart ischemic. The coronary artery is very small and can be difficult to cannulate. For example, the cannula may dislodge from the artery while it is being sutured into the coronary artery. The cannula may also dislodge if the knot is not secure around the head of the cannula when adjusting the various tension parameters of the right ventricular wall. It is possible, however, to recannulate the coronary artery by carefully cutting off the previous knot, reinserting the cannula, and resuturing it while the wall is still mounted and perfused.

Perfusion defects may occur by improper cannulation or if the small bifurcating vessel off the right coronary is insufficiently clamped or tied. Small nicks in the right coronary arteries near the cannula may also cause reduced performance. If a leak can be located, it may be possible to clamp the hole closed using a microvascular serrefine clamp.

Although generally a stable preparation, the right ventricular wall may develop arrhythmias. This may be due in part to insufficiently trimming off papillaries or septal tissue from the right wall. These tissues may be trimmed off while the heart is being perfused using spring scissors and fine tipped curved forceps. Arrhythmias may develop if perfusion temperatures exceed 37°C, or if there are contaminants in the perfusate or perfusion lines.

It is important to clean the tubing at the end of each working day with 0.1 N HCl and 70% ethanol for at least 5 min each, followed by pumping de-ionized water through the system. Bacterial contamination can be a serious detriment to heart performance, particularly at the lower flow rates employed here. Tubing should be replaced completely in the entire perfusion system on at least a bimonthly basis. All other nonmetal fittings and stopcocks should be occasionally soaked overnight in 0.1 N HCl or replaced. Metal parts in the perfusion system must be made of corrosion-proof metal, such as high quality stainless steel for clamps, and platinum or gold for stimulating electrodes. Surfaces can be coated with a nontoxic plastic or enamel coating for additional protection.

Since peristaltic tubing wears with use, it is important to calibrate pump out-flow through the cannula at least once a week. Decreased flow rates can reduce performance and lead to inconsistent results.

2.5.   Special Experimental Conditions

2.5.1.   Ischemia reperfusion

The right ventricular wall preparation is an excellent model for ischemia reperfusion. Ischemia is accomplished by turning off the peristaltic pump and covering the apparatus with a Plexiglas hood (Figure 1). Nitrogen is bubbled in an internal hot water bath to maintain temperature and humidity. The ischemic environment must be moist, to prevent dehydration of the ventricle, during periods of no/low flow. Temperature is monitored by a digital thermometer probe inserted in the top of the Plexiglas hood at the exact height of the heart. The heated water bath is regulated with a temperature feedback controller. Nitrogen (or any inert gas) is used to bubble the water bath. Reperfusion is initiated by turning on the peristaltic pump and initiating flow at 37°C. The chamber hood is removed to parallel pre-ischemic conditions.

2.5.2. Hypoxia reoxygenation

The procedure for hypoxia is similar to that of ischemia, except that the flow to the ventricle is maintained and the perfusate is changed to an oxygen-depleted solution for the period of hypoxia. The hypoxic solution should have been previously bubbled with an inert gas to exclude oxygen. It is then pumped through a second set of perfusion lines, to calibrate perfusate temperature, just prior to the hypoxic insult to the heart. Flow is initiated by switching stopcock direction.

2.5.3. Drug delivery

In order to test the effect of a drug on the right ventricular wall, it is important to have two or more separate perfusion lines installed within the system, as well as a 3- or 4-way stopcock near the cannula. Prior to drug delivery, the drug-containing solution must be allowed to pump freely through the auxiliary perfusion lines to equilibrate perfusate temperature. Changing the position of the stopcock can then allow infusion of the perfusate containing the drug.

In summary, the isolated, coronary-perfused right ventricular wall preparation is an excellent choice as a model in which to study cardiac performance. In some cases, it offers distinct advantages over the other cardiac preparations available while still showing the same basic physiological and pathological responses. However, in some experimental settings, it may not be the optimal method of choice. The researcher must be fully aware of the potential benefits and pitfalls of the technique in order to optimize the results generated.

Acknowledgments

This work was supported by the Heart and Stroke Foundation of Manitoba. Hamid Massaeli is a trainee of the Heart and Stroke Foundation of Canada. Grant N. Pierce is a scientist of the Medical Research Council of Canada.

References

1. Langer, G. A. and Brady, A. J., The effects of temperature upon contraction and ionic exchange in rabbit ventricular myocardium: relation to control of active state, *J. Gen. Physiol.*, 52, 682, 1968.
2. Pierce, G. N., Rich, T. L., and Langer, G. A., Transsarcolemmal Ca^{2+} movements associated with contraction of the rabbit right ventricular wall, *Circ. Res.*, 61, 805, 1987.
3. Meng, H. and Pierce, G. N., Protective effects of 5-(N,N-dimethyl) amiloride on ischemia-reperfusion injury in hearts, *Am. J. Physiol.*, 258, H1615, 1990.

4. Meng, H., Lonsberry, B. B., and Pierce, G. N., Influence of perfusate pH on the post-ischemic recovery of cardiac contractile function: involvement of sodium-hydrogen exchange, *J. Pharmacol. Exp. Ther.*, 258, 772, 1991.

5. Meng, H. and Pierce, G. N., Involvement of sodium in the protective effect of 5-(N,N-dimethyl) amiloride (DMA) on ischemia-reperfusion injury in isolated rat heart, *J. Pharmacol. Exp. Ther.*, 256, 1094, 1991.

6. Meng, H., Maddaford, T. G., and Pierce, G. N., The effect of amiloride and several selected analogues on post-ischemic recovery of cardiac contractile function, *Am. J. Physiol.*, 264, H1831, 1993.

7. Pierce, G. N., Cole, W. C., Liu, K., Massaeli, H., Maddaford, T. G., Chen, Y. G., McPherson, C. D., Jain, S., and Sontag, D., Modulation of cardiac performance by amiloride and several selected derivatives of amiloride, *J. Pharmacol. Exp. Ther.*, 265, 1280, 1993.

8. McPherson, C. D., Pierce, G. N., and Cole, W. C., Ischemic cardioprotection by ATP-sensitive K^+ channels involves high-energy phosphate preservation, *Am. J. Physiol.*, 265, H1809, 1993.

9. Panagiotopoulos, S., Daly, M. J., and Nayler, W. G., Effect of acidosis and alkalosis on postischemic Ca^{2+} gain in isolated rat heart, *Am. J. Physiol.*, 258, H821, 1990.

10. Moffat, M. P., Karmazyn, M., and Ferrier, G. R., Prostaglandin involvement in hypersensitivity of ischemic hearts to arrhythmogenic influence of ouabain, *Am. J. Physiol.*, 249, 1985.

11. Kim, D.-H., Akera, T., and Kennedy, R. H., Ischemia-induced enhancement of digitalis sensitivity in isolated guinea-pig heart, *J. Pharmacol. Exp. Ther.*, 226, 335, 1983.

12. Gupta, M., Makino, N., Kaneko, M., and Dhalla, N. S., Cardiac sarcolemma as a possible site of action of caffeine in rat heart, *J. Pharmacol. Exp. Ther.*, 255, 1188, 1990.

13. Grinwald, P. M. and Brosnahan, C., Sodium imbalance as a cause of calcium overload in post-hypoxic reoxygenation injury, *J. Mol. Cell. Cardiol.*, 19, 487, 1987.

14. Weiss, J., Couper, G. S., Hiltbrand, B., and Shine, K. I., Role of acidosis in early contractile dysfunction during ischemia: evidence from pH_o measurements, *Am. J. Physiol.*, 247, H760, 1984.

15. Shine, K. I., Douglas, A. M., and Ricchiuti, N. V., Calcium, strontium, and barium movements during ischemia and reperfusion in rabbit ventricle, *Circ. Res.*, 43, 712, 1978.

16. Mitani, A., Kinoshita, K., Fukamachi, K., Sakamoto, M., Kurisu, K., Tsuruhara, Y., Fukumura, F., Nakashima, A., and Tokunaga, K., Effects of glibenclamide and nicorandil on cardiac function during ischemia and reperfusion in isolated perfused rat hearts, *Am. J. Physiol.*, 261, H1864, 1991.

17. Karmazyn, M., Amiloride enhances postischemic ventricular recovery: possible role of Na^+-H^+ exchange, *Am. J. Physiol.*, 255, H608, 1988.

18. Moffat, M. P. and Karmazyn, M., Protective effects of the potent Na^+/H^+ exchange inhibitor methylisobutyl amiloride against post-ischemic contractile dysfunction in rat and guinea-pig hearts, *J. Mol. Cell. Cardiol.*, 25, 959, 1993.

19. Cole, W. C., McPherson, C. D., and Sontag, D., ATP-regulated K^+ channels protect the myocardium against ischemia/reperfusion damage, *Circ. Res.*, 69, 571, 1991.
20. Backx, P. H. and Ter Keurs, H. E. D. J., The fluorescent properties of rat cardiac trabeculae loaded with Fura-2 salt, *Am. J. Physiol*, 264, H1098, 1993.

Index

Printed and bound by CPI Group (UK) Ltd, Croydon, CR0 4YY

17/10/2024

01775691-0003